W9-BSL-697

# CALORIES

# DON'T

# COUNT

BY

HERMAN TALLER,

M.D.

NEW YORK

SIMON AND SCHUSTER    1961

All rights reserved
including the right of reproduction
in whole or in part in any form
Copyright © 1961 by Herman Taller
Published by Simon and Schuster, Inc.
Rockefeller Center, 630 Fifth Avenue
New York 20, N. Y.

THIRTEENTH PRINTING

Library of Congress Catalog Card Number: 61–12849
Manufactured in the United States of America

*To my dear parents,*
*Samuel and Matilda*
*And to my beloved children,*
*Myron and Monette*

# CONTENTS

# PREFACE

Excess fat, recognized throughout the ages as an ugly, disfiguring thing, has only recently been recognized as something else. Over the last few decades physicians, scientists and large portions of the public at large have come to understand that excess fat is a serious threat to health. There is no longer any question that obesity is a disease. It is a disease and sometimes a grave one.

But agreement about obesity stops just there. Until now there has been no agreement on how to treat this evil. There have been dozens of theories, hundreds of fads, some popular, some obscure, but all joined by a single point: They didn't work. For all the theories, formulas and fads, obesity, like its victims, has become more and more widespread every year. Modern medicine, despite all the wonders it works with devastating ailments, has not been able to help most fat people grow slim.

The concept this book advances is revolutionary. Perhaps all I need say in support of my new nutrition principle is that it works. It has been tested in medical laboratories and among large numbers of patients. There have been no failures, nor can there be any when the principle is properly applied. For this new principle is based on new knowledge—a medical breakthrough, so to speak. Before proceeding, I think it is wise to warn you that this break-through is so dramatic that it will probably invalidate all you know, or think you know, about the cause and the treatment of obesity.

What is needed now is a vast program of re-education, organized on two levels. First, physicians must be re-educated in all the areas of the world where obesity is a problem. For this there are medical journals, which have published and are publishing the scientific explanation of this breakthrough. Such papers, couched in technical terminology, written by scientists for scientists, are lost on the general public.

It is my hope that this book will *not* be lost on the general public. It is written for the public. For, just as physicians are now being re-educated, so the public must learn to discard large quantities of erroneous information that have been taught and absorbed in good faith over the years. The public, then, must re-educate itself on the whole problem of obesity. Entrenched ideas die hard, and I suspect that it may be a long process.

To begin your re-education, there are certain points about this book and its author which I want to stress. I am a physician with a good many years of experience behind me. I would no more offer an untested program to the public than I would offer an untested program to a patient who walked into my office filled with faith that I would do the right thing to the best of my ability and knowledge. I would not have written this book, nor have prescribed the new nutrition principle to my patients, if

I were not sure that it was entirely safe and entirely effective. I would not have prepared papers for other physicians to study if I did not possess an imposing body of evidence.

I do not assert that we now know everything about obesity. Of course we don't. We don't know everything about infections either. But we can cure infections, almost all of them. So now we can successfully treat victims of obesity, almost all of them, too.

I want you to get the most that you possibly can out of this book and out of the program it explains for you. *Calories Don't Count* begins with an explanation of how I first became interested in obesity and then proceeds to a brief history of man's continuing, unsuccessful battle against excess fat over the centuries. After considering in detail the dangers obesity presents and re-examining, in the light of current knowledge, fads and fallacies—including that prize of all fallacies, the low-calorie diet—it discusses the role of food and the causes of obesity.

It is not necessary for you to understand a cause to understand a treatment. Penicillin works as well for infants as it does for learned physicians. But I do hope you make an effort to grasp the scientific considerations behind my new nutrition principle. You can, if you wish, skip the theory and proceed directly to the chapter which tells you what to do. But once you see how effectively this principle works, you will probably want to follow it for the rest of your life. With that in mind, I suggest that learning why the principle does work makes sense.

11

More than 95 per cent of all obese people are fat because of a disturbance which this principle counteracts. However, there does exist that 5 per cent, that one person in twenty, whose obesity probably stems from a glandular condition. Perhaps, before putting my principle into practice for yourself, you may want to visit your personal physician to make sure that you are among the 95 per cent that can be helped. It is a good idea to undergo a complete physical examination before undertaking the new program. This book can, and I hope does, explain for you just what the program is and how to follow it. But it cannot examine you to make certain your glands are functioning normally. Only your physician can do that, and he will be glad to.

It is conceivable that your physician may not yet know of the new principle. Physicians are busy men; even the most dedicated cannot keep up with all the latest research in all the varied fields of medicine. And, as I say, this principle is based on recent research.

If he has not heard of it, you may, obviously, refer him to this book. In addition he also might want to consult technical papers, published by myself and by the late Dr. Alfred Pennington before me, which are available in medical reference libraries. All of us in medicine have only recently begun to learn about the role played by carbohydrates in obesity and the role played by substances called polyunsaturated fatty acids in the treatment of obesity. The necessary re-education, on the level of physician and on the level of patient, has only begun.

With this book, *you* are ready to begin. Drop your old

prejudices, theories and superstitions of obesity, and drop them cheerfully. After all, you have nothing to lose but your girth.

HERMAN TALLER, M.D., F.A.C.O.G., F.I.C.S.
Brooklyn, New York
June 1961

# CHAPTER ONE

# I EAT FAT—
# AND GROW THIN

THIS BOOK IS THE STORY of a search. It was a search I pursued for a long time, as other medical research workers had before me, but what makes this particular story exciting is that the search was not fruitless. It led to a discovery. I have found out what makes most people fat.

More than that, I've found a way for most fat people to reduce, a way which probably contradicts almost everything you've heard about reducing but which is as certain and exact as the science of chemistry. For that is precisely the basis of this new nutrition principle—the biochemistry of the human body.

There is no magic involved, there are no tricks, no injections, no pills. By following this principle you can eat as much as anyone could reasonably want. You can forget about calories. Since under this principle you will lose fat, not muscle or other vital body substance, you reduce without growing gaunt-necked or flabby-armed. To some of my patients, who came to me after years of unsuccessful dieting, the principle has seemed to be a miracle. It isn't, of course. It is simply one more instance of the advance of science. It has not been discovered until now because, frankly, until now none of us—not doctors, nor chemists, nor other nutrition experts—knew enough about the biochemistry of the body.

Later on, we can go into this principle in detail so that you can understand, just as my patients do, what foods are the fat producers and why. I'll explain the wide range of foods you can eat, the large quantities you can have, the things specifically to avoid. But for now I'd like to tell you about my search, how it started, where it took me and how it came to such a happy ending. For what has been a happy ending for me can become one for you as well, if you adopt this simple principle and follow it carefully.

I had been a fat man all my life. I stand 5 feet 10½ inches and at one time I weighed 265 pounds. From boyhood I was always chubby, and an unpleasant memory that remains with me is that I was often called "Fat" or "Fatty" as a child. Obesity ran in my family. My brother was fat and my sister was fat. There didn't seem to be anything that we could do about our fat but accept it. As a matter of fact, at the time there *was* nothing else we could do.

When I entered medical school at the University of Pavia in Italy, I asked physicians about "diets" and studied any number of medical papers on nutrition. There were theories by the dozen, but, from my point of view, one thing was wrong with all of them. Not one worked for me.

At Pavia everyone ate great quantities of spaghetti. Most of the other students ate spaghetti and kept their weight. I felt I had only to look at a platter of spaghetti to gain. As much as I could avoid eating spaghetti and exist in Italy, I did. All through medical school I was hungry.

I tried diets on which I ate nothing but fresh fruits. I'd lose a few pounds that way, but then when I went off the diet I'd gain back what I had lost and more. Why did I go off these diets? On a steady routine of fruits, I became weak and nervous. Fruits were not enough to sustain me.

I tried limiting my food to milk and vegetables. For an entire month, that was all I ate. At the end of the month I found I had gained three pounds.

I tried a protein diet, concentrating on meats and fish. This turned out to be just one more way for me to gain weight.

At the end of my career in medical school, I weighed 35 pounds more than I had when I matriculated. Besides, as I say, I had been hungry most of the time. You've heard the myth about the jolly fat man. I was a hungry fat man and I assure you there was nothing jolly about my hunger or my being fat. (In fact, I've treated enough fat people to be absolutely certain there is nothing jolly about *anybody's* being fat.)

By the time I graduated from Pavia, shortly before

17

World War II erupted, the Chilean government had sent word that their country was in serious need of physicians. I realized that my own native land, Roumania, would soon be overrun by Nazis, so I went halfway round the world and began to practice among poor people in a small government clinic in Chile. It was called St. Vincent de Paul Hospital.

Living in Chile, I encountered an entirely different diet from the sort I had known as a child and at medical school in Italy. Black beans were the staple; they are to Chile what spaghetti is to Italy. But whether it was beans or spaghetti or almost anything else, the effect always seemed to be the same: On my frame, the food turned to fat.

Of course I was concerned. One day I mentioned my feelings to Dr. Edwin Reed, who was chief of the medical division of the South American Shipping Company.

"I think I have an idea," Dr. Reed said.

"What is it?"

"Become a ship's doctor," Dr. Reed said. "Come to work for me. Aboard a ship, you'll be able to follow a strict nutrition pattern, a strict diet. That way you should be able to control your weight."

I accepted his offer and a week later sailed from Chile to Ecuador aboard the passenger ship *Mapocho*. I spoke six languages—French, Spanish, Portuguese, Italian, German and Roumanian—and I played bridge, so I had no trouble making friends. It was comfortable settling down to the routine of a ship's doctor, but, for me at least, it was fattening. At sea as on land, I could find no method of satisfying my nutritional needs that did not also make me gain weight. I was not to find even the beginnings of the new nutrition principle until years later when I was practicing in the United States.

Only a fortunate accident brought me to the United States and the position where I could start investigations into the biochemistry of the human body. The physician on the *Copiapó*, which sailed regularly from Valparaiso to New York, suddenly became ill and I was asked to replace him. As I said, I spoke six languages—but not English. I had never been to America. Naturally, the prospect of seeing New York was very exciting. I accepted the offer readily.

It was then that a new life started. I learned English, took an internship and residency in an outstanding Brooklyn hospital and opened practice as an obstetrician and gynecologist. For a time my principal interest was natural childbirth. But I could never quite forget the problem of obesity.

For one thing, as my weight constantly grew, clothing was expensive. I seemed to be constantly buying new suits, new shirts, new topcoats. Then, too, in supervising the regimen of pregnant women, I was constantly prescribing diets, which must have made some of my patients wonder. After all, here was a very heavy physician advising them how to control their weight.

Of course, I discussed weight control with other physicians. I mentioned my own experiments with diets, and

19

some of them hinted that I must have "cheated," eaten on the sly, admitting to no one, perhaps not even to myself, what I had been doing. Other physicians who had weight problems themselves simply shrugged. The more I discussed weight, the more questions I asked, the more surely I was convinced that there simply were no answers in the existing body of medical knowledge.

Once, to another physician who seemed particularly certain that I was cheating, I proposed an interesting vacation test. We would go away together for ten days, stay in each other's company continually, eat and drink the same things and check the results. He accepted, and we went off to a resort. I followed what was then the accepted method of weight control: a low-calorie diet. I concentrated on salads, which I now know was a mistake, ate fat sparingly, another mistake, and, since this was a vacation, drank a cocktail each night before dinner. My physician friend, who was slim, did the same. At the end of the vacation, he had lost a pound or two and I had gained nine pounds. "I don't understand it," he said as we drove back to New York. Neither did I.

I don't mean to suggest that a crash diet, a semistarvation program, would not work for me. Whenever I tried one I did lose some poundage. But then, afterward, I invariably gained back more than I had lost. Besides, there were disturbing side effects to crash programs, specifically fatigue and irritability. What I do suggest, in fact what I do know, is that as recently as ten years ago no weight-reduction program which one could sustain would succeed for an individual who was innately inclined toward obesity.

In 1955, you may remember, doctors were becoming very interested in cholesterol, a fatlike substance found in the blood stream, and its relationship to coronary disease. At the time there seemed to be some connection between obesity and cholesterol, and so, being heavy, I took a cholesterol test myself. It was a simple test; it just involves taking a minute quantity of blood. My cholesterol count turned out to be above 350, which is to say 350 milligrams for every 100 cubic centimeters of blood serum. A normal cholesterol count was then considered to be 225. Apparently I had something to worry about.

"I want you to try something," said the researcher who had taken my blood. He showed me an oily substance and then, to demonstrate that it was harmless, drank some of it himself.

"What is it?" I asked.

"I'm not ready to tell you," the investigator said.

I sampled his potion. It was not delicious, but it was palatable. With my high cholesterol level, I was willing to experiment, so I began drinking three ounces of the mystery substance daily. (Recently developed capsules have made the routine easier.) And I suggested that a few physicians I knew, who were concerned about their cholesterol levels, do the same. Meanwhile, I was to report for cholesterol-level tests every two weeks.

As the researcher had anticipated, my cholesterol level began to drop. But I also began to lose weight. A colleague was the first to point this out.

"Impossible," I said. "In addition to my regular meals, I'm taking in this oil which is very high in calories. I'm taking in five thousand calories a day."

"You're losing weight," he insisted.

Sure enough, within two or three weeks I noticed that I was fastening my belt on a tighter notch. Here I was, eating margarine, drinking oil, and losing weight.

Some physician friends of mine became concerned and spoke to me about it. "Are you certain you're all right?" they asked.

"I feel fine," I said, for I actually felt much better than I had. Still, they looked at me and shook their heads.

When I found out what the substance was—technically, a polyunsaturated fatty acid—I headed for the library of the Kings County Medical Society. I wanted to know what was happening to my own biochemistry, what it meant to the biochemistry of others, what it meant to all the theories of weight gain and weight loss.

Try to imagine how I felt. I was a trained physician who, for professional and personal reasons, had become unusually conversant with nutritional theories. For decades I had read what was accepted as an unshakable rule: To lose weight, cut calories. Now, by increasing calories, I was losing weight. Was this some fluke? Would what worked for me work for others? Would it work for my patients? And if it did work, why did it work? Could it be,

22

I asked myself, that calories don't count? Could I say to my patients, "Don't count calories"?

With hope and a feeling of excitement, I began spending all my spare time in the medical library. In the index there, I looked for everything that existed on obesity and metabolism. I can tell you that it was a discouraging time. Nearly all of the papers and books I read presumed that calories did count. Then, finally, I found what was to be the beginning of my own work.

In the *Journal of the Medical Society of Delaware* for April 1951 appeared an article entitled "The Use of Fat in a Weight-Reducing Diet." The author was the late Dr. Alfred W. Pennington. I read the title two or three times, for it described what was happening to me. Then, as I went on, I saw this paragraph:

> Contrary to the claims of the low-calorie school of thought, low-calorie diets have failed under the most rigid experimental conditions. Low-calorie diets, based on the principle of caloric requirements, are crudely devised in the service of simplicity. There are fat people, plenty of them, who are actually starving.

When Dr. Pennington prepared this paper in 1951, little was known of the difference between saturated and unsaturated fatty acids, a point which is significant, if technical, and which we shall consider at length in succeeding chapters. But he had the first glimmer, the first specific evidence, I had found to explain what was happening to me. In addition to asserting that low-calorie diets did not assure weight loss, Dr. Pennington went on to assert that certain fats did.

All my training told me that Dr. Pennington must be in error. Yet my own body seemed to be telling me he was correct. He wrote that the calorie theory presumed "if a person eats less than his caloric requirement, he will lose weight; and if the predictions of the calculator are not fulfilled, the patient is suspected of being a glutton on the sly." I knew, from sad experience, that this was an accurate description.

Then I encountered a key sentence of explanation: *"The ability of tissues to oxidize fat is, in contrast to carbohydrates, unlimited."* "Oxidize" means to burn up. Your body burns up food to create the energy you need through the process of oxidization. Dr. Pennington was making an exciting point. The body, he was maintaining, can burn up an unlimited amount of fat, can transform an unlimited amount of fat into energy. If you burn all the fat you eat, there is not going to be any fat left. Fat, then, is not going to make you gain weight, provided you take sufficient exercise. (This was brilliant original research, but later it was to be modified somewhat.)

But what about carbohydrates? Here, Dr. Pennington had found, the chemistry of the body was limited. The body could burn only a certain quantity of carbohydrates, the exact quantity varying with the individual. What happens to the carbohydrates that aren't burned? The body stores them. And how does the body store them? As fat. In the case of men the body concentrates excess fat about the stomach, as "middle-age spread," and at the back of the

24

neck, and in the case of women it concentrates excess fat on the buttocks, the upper arms, the upper legs and the breasts, as well as on the abdomen.

Some people may think of carbohydrates only as obvious sugars and starches, as candy and potatoes. But actually most vegetables are largely carbohydrate. The salads I had eaten on vacation—while passing up dressing—were carbohydrates. The fruits I had eaten in medical school were carbohydrates. I do not think it is going too far to say that Dr. Pennington's work struck me as revolutionary.

While I was considering and studying Dr. Pennington's paper, other physicians continued to worry about my weight loss. The drop was steady and dramatic and they feared that I was suffering from the beginnings of some wasting illness. I disregarded everybody, because my index was my own health. I knew how I was feeling. A chronic stuffy nose was getting better. My complexion was improving, and over eight months I lost a total of 65 pounds. I was not a thin man at 200, but I was far thinner, and far happier, than I had been for years.

I started a correspondence with Dr. Pennington while I was taking the oil, losing weight and making certain diet modifications of my own. I remember something this distinguished scientist said in a letter to me. "Of low-calorie diets there are many," Dr. Pennington wrote, "but of obese people who have solved their problem there are very few."

I knew then what my mission was. It was to proceed

from Dr. Pennington's beginnings, to forget low-calorie diets and to march forward toward a program that would solve the problems of obese people, even as my own elementary program was so happily solving mine.

# CHAPTER TWO

# CENTURIES

# OF FAT

THERE IS A FORWARD FLOW to medical research. There is no other area in which human progress and human interdependence is more marked. If Louis Pasteur had not formulated the germ theory of disease, Sir Alexander Fleming would probably not have discovered penicillin. He could not have been looking for an antibiotic had he not known there were microbes to be killed. So, conceivably, penicillin might have been dismissed as just another insignificant mold.

The last hundred years have been bountiful with medical discoveries. Most of us know the magnificent strides that have been taken in the control of smallpox, yellow fever, scores of other ailments and, more recently, a wide variety of infections, polio and tuberculosis. With all this, why, you may wonder, had so little been done on the problem of excess fat?

One answer is that only recently has fat been traced as a contributory factor to many ailments and to many early deaths. Another answer may be that compared say, to cholera, obesity is not a very dramatic disease. Cholera kills quickly. Fat kills as surely as cholera does, but slowly, over a long period of years. I am going to present evidence that should terminate any doubts you may have about the advisability of weight reduction. But for the moment I want to explain just where medical scientists stood when Dr. Pennington presented his paper—where we stood and how we had got there.

Actually, the first high-fat diet was proposed a century ago. It was proposed, it was tested on a very limited basis, and it seemed to work. Then it was promptly forgotten.

William Banting, who published "The Banting Diet" in 1863, was the patient of an English ear surgeon named William Harvey. Banting was a corpulent, slightly deaf man of sixty, with an earache.

Harvey had been in Paris listening to lectures by Claude Bernard, a prominent French scientist, who had developed a new theory of biochemistry. The liver, Bernard believed, secreted not only bile but a peculiar substance, chemically allied to sugar and starches, which Bernard named glucose.

Harvey not only listened; he wondered, and he began to formulate a theory himself. He started with two facts:

1. An animal diet—that is, a diet composed exclusively of meats—checked the secretion of diabetic urine.

2. A diet high in sugar and starch had, in tests, fattened certain farm animals.

28

Diabetes was a fascination of Harvey's. Bernard's theory had started him thinking about the relationship between sugars, starches and fats. Now, with his two facts, he reached a tentative conclusion. Excessive weight, he decided, contributed toward diabetes; obesity in itself might not start diabetes, but if there was a tendency toward the disease obesity could very well tip the scales, so to speak. Next, Harvey experimented and found that diabetics seemed to be helped by a diet that was low in sugar and starch and high in protein.

He was puzzling over carbohydrate metabolism when William Banting walked into his office, holding one ear.

After a careful examination, Harvey found nothing organically wrong with William Banting's ear. There was no evidence of disease, no sign of infection. Harvey looked at his portly patient and pondered whether it might not be fat that was causing the earache. Excessive fat, he believed, could be creating pressure on Banting's eustachian tube. This canal, which runs from the middle ear inward, is extremely sensitive.

Still experimenting, Harvey prescribed an unorthodox diet for Banting, consisting of venison, poultry and fish but devoid of sugars and starches. (He did allow Banting limited amounts of alcoholic drinks, on the mistaken notion that the body eliminates alcohol completely, the way it eliminates water.)

A year later William Banting was 46 pounds lighter. Since he had been allowed up to 24 ounces of meat and fish a day, and since he liked these foods, he was quite

29

cheerful. His earache was gone and his hearing was fully restored. Gratified, Banting published his "diet" on his own.

As often happens in such cases, medical authorities were skeptical. In fact, they were more than skeptical. They ridiculed both Banting and Harvey. Since the diet had not appeared in a medical publication, it was attacked as "unscientific." Some described it as freakish. Others insisted that following the Banting diet was so expensive that it was not practical.

Still there was the nagging question of results. The diet had worked for Banting, and letters which Banting received indicated that it worked for others as well. Such practical success had to be explained and a Dr. Neimeyer of Stuttgart, Germany, obligingly offered a reason. Proteins, he said, could not be converted into body fat, but both carbohydrates and fats could be. In other words, he was advocating what would now be called a high-protein, low-carbohydrate diet. This modified Banting Diet actually found its way into standard textbooks some eighty years ago. Meanwhile Harvey, his brief adventure into nutrition concluded, went back to ear surgery, but not before publishing a book on general health, in which he recanted his original theory. He supported the Neimeyer high-protein approach, leaving Banting pretty much alone in support of fat.

In the modified Banting diets that followed, the high-protein principle became more and more firmly established and dietary fat intake was increasingly restricted.

In retrospect, it seems unfortunate that with research workers so close to a real understanding of the role fat plays in weight loss, there was this sudden shift in emphasis from fat to protein. In the light of present-day knowledge, Harvey's original diet was the most effective in principle, and it would have been more so had he reduced the allowable alcohol intake. But progress is not a steady, measurable thing. From the diet William Banting followed, medical science marched backward for a time. Harvey's major error was his decision not to pursue his experimentation further.

As the twentieth century began, most physicians agreed that obesity was caused by insufficient oxidation of fat. This was an approach through metabolism, an approach which maintained that the biochemistry of some was not geared to burn enough fat. This theory is wrong and, in reality, is only half a theory. It considers the body's burning of fat, but ignores a critical point. What about the body's formation of fat? Early in the twentieth century, no physician could have given you a reasonable answer.

Later the general view changed. By 1930, doctors were discounting metabolic theories and concentrating instead on faulty eating habits. Here is where calories came in. If the body took in more calories, these physicians believed, the extra calories would be converted into fat. Many still hold to this belief. Entrenched medical theories, however erroneous, are a long time in dying.

31

What's wrong with the calorie theory? As you remember, Dr. Pennington discovered that the body can burn unlimited amounts of fat, but only limited amounts of carbohydrates. With his discovery, it became evident that it was not the quantity of food a person ate as much as the *types* of food he ate that mattered. For in the biochemistry of the body all calories are not the same. To say that a specific number of calories will make you fat is as silly as it is to say that a certain number of microbes will make you sick. What kind of calories? What kind of microbes?

The caloric theory became the rage in America. Numberless books were published. Small "calorie counters" were printed. Millions of people read the books, counted their calories and grew fatter and fatter. Further, the calorie theory was, in a sense, quite cruel. If you grew fat while limiting your calories, something was clearly wrong. It couldn't be the theory, most people decided. So, if it wasn't the theory, it had to be you.

Were you really counting all your calories? Did you count that 2 A.M. trip to the refrigerator? Did you count that second martini? What about the snack you had at three in the afternoon? Protest as you would, no one believed you. Certainly you knew that at 2 A.M. you had been asleep, that you hadn't had a second martini, and that at three in the afternoon you were busy with your work. But nobody else did. Other people winked or grinned, and you felt miserable. In my practice I have encountered numerous cases in which patients were acutely depressed by their husbands' conviction that they were

32

cheating on calories. It can create a serious disturbance within the home.

Oddly enough, at the height of the calorie craze further experiments were taking place which proved the theory false. A New York physician, Blake F. Donaldson, introduced a high-calorie diet at one hospital with considerable success. Dr. Donaldson treated obese patients with diets consisting of up to 24 ounces of meat a day, fully one fourth of them fat. Imagine the reaction of the antifat faddists when Dr. Donaldson's patients lost weight. Oh, the protein was acceptable, the faddists said, but how to explain the fat?

Harvey had been close to an explanation years before, but physicians and scientists were so deeply involved in the calorie theory that many were determined to protect it at all costs—even, it seems, logic. The diet was monotonous, one scientist said, so what actually had happened was that patients had eaten less than before, perhaps without realizing they were cutting down. Eating fat makes you want less food, someone else said, advancing the same idea. But evidence refuted both these points. Without much encouragement, these patients ate copiously. Most of them liked to eat and now they had a physician's hearty permission to eat as much as they wanted. In many cases they ate more than they ever had before. Still they lost weight.

It is hardly a secret that in these times strong commercial pressures affect nutritional beliefs. Commercial manufacturers of low-calorie foods base all their advertising on the low-calorie theory. All of us are, to some degree, affected by the advertising that we see. In spite of Dr. Donaldson's evidence, the calorie theory persisted.

But even as Dr. Donaldson worked, there was strong evidence from the Arctic Circle that calories didn't count. Vilhjalmur Stefansson, the explorer, had traveled to the Arctic early in the century and had lived among the Eskimos and studied their ways, which were then unknown to most of the outside world. He paid particularly close attention to what the Eskimos ate. Stefansson was not a missionary or a trader. He was simply an observer. He did not go north to sell or to teach. He went north to learn.

The Eskimos, he saw, were a strong, healthy race and they subsisted on a diet which consisted largely of meat and animal and marine fat. The fat included great quantities of whale blubber. Yet the Eskimos did not suffer from obesity.

Stefansson, after years of careful study, reasoned that man had been a hunting creature originally and had lived entirely by the meat and fat of fish and animals. Only later did man start growing his own foods, the foods that are so heavily carbohydrate.

Historians feel that the shift from the hunters' diet to the agricultural diet took place less than fifteen thousand years ago in China, five thousand years ago in Greece and Italy, and only two thousand years ago in England. (Julius Caesar saw Belgic settlers introducing agriculture to Britons for the first time.)

"If meat needs carbohydrate and other vegetable additions to make it wholesome," Stefansson wrote later, "then the poor Eskimos were not eating healthfully . . . they should have been in a wretched state. On the contrary, they seemed to me the healthiest people I had ever lived with." (It is interesting to note that while the Eskimo does not eat citrus fruit in his usual diet, investigation revealed that the vitamin-C content in an average Eskimo's blood was much higher than that of the average Canadian, who was eating a "normal" diet and living in a similar climate.)

When Stefansson returned to the United States and published his conclusions, the book was called a wide variety of things. "Controversial" was mild. "Fantastic" was more common. Stefansson, in addition to reporting the high-fat diet he had seen in the Arctic, advocated its general use. By now, of course, he has brilliantly answered all those who called him a fraud when he first returned from the Far North. Still following a high-fat, high-protein diet, he is in excellent health—and in his eighties.

What existed before the work of Dr. Pennington, then, was conflict and a puzzle. No one, least of all myself, would dispute the concept that led to the calorie fad. Any person will lose weight when he burns up more energy than he eats. This is a simple chemical law. Why, then, didn't a low-calorie diet work? Why did people lose weight on high-calorie, high-fat diets? What was needed was a whole series of complex studies of energy balance within the human body.

Medical researchers spent years wrestling with these

questions. Some of what they found appeared to conflict with other things they had found. It was a long, difficult, painstaking job before Dr. Pennington, reviewing the whole mass of complicated data, began to resolve it into a clear-cut pattern. He later told me that it was with considerable confidence that he rose before a medical convention to deliver this verdict: "Obesity is due to excessive intake of carbohydrates, plus a disturbance in metabolism due to a physiological (organic) disturbance of the body." (Again, a brilliant point, but one that now can be carried further.)

You now have, as I had, the first clue to weight control. Limit your intake of carbohydrates. But what is the physiological disturbance? Does this mean that something is wrong with your system if you're fat? Does it mean that you have some sort of sickness? The answer is that something is wrong with one of your body functions. This function is a part of the over-all metabolism of the human body.

In the process of breaking down a carbohydrate, say a piece of bread, the body goes through many chemical steps, one of which is the formation of a substance called pyruvic acid. Now, if your body is functioning well, it burns pyruvic acid for energy and, in the process, creates carbon dioxide and water. You rid yourself of the carbon dioxide in breath and of the water in urine. So, ideally, there is no excess fat created.

But many obese people seem unable to burn pyruvic

36

acid at a reasonable rate. What happens in their systems is quite different and, to them, quite distressing, although they cannot feel it happening.

Through another complicated process, the faulty system turns pyruvic acid into other substances called fatty acids, which in turn combine with glycerol to form glycerides. The chemistry may not be important to you, but the results should be. Glycerides—specifically, triglycerides—are the greatest culprits in making people fat.

This is about as far as Pennington went, but it was far enough—too far, perhaps, for some conservatives. His concept of human biochemistry was strange and revolutionary, but there was one overwhelming argument for it: The concept fit the facts. Harvey's diet had been based on very few facts. The science of physiology, when Harvey lived, was hardly a science at all. It was largely guesswork. Dr. Donaldson's treatment was based on more evidence, but still no one could then have told you why the treatment worked, only that it did work. Perhaps this is why it was not adopted more widely.

But in the light of Pennington's work, one could assert with absolute certainty that the calorie theory had no scientific basis whatsoever. It is merely a vague sort of treatment, like bed rest for a cold. When it works, it usually functions through the process of semistarvation. It is a subnutritional diet; the body does not get enough of what it needs. When a low-calorie diet is called a "crash diet," the term is perfect. A low-calorie diet causes a physical crash and can, carried to extremes, prove to be fatal. Many a public figure has been killed by crash diets within the last few years.

When a diet includes unrestricted quantities of calories, the degree to which carbohydrates must be restricted varies with individuals. The capacity of individuals to convert carbohydrates into energy, carbon dioxide and water is quite important here, and this, like any individual function, is not the same in different people. I mention this lest you suddenly decide simply to eliminate all carbohydrates from your own diet. Wait until you learn more. What I have evolved from the work of Pennington and others, and from my own research, is a new nutrition principle which touches your entire way of life. Until you grasp all of the principle, it would be unwise to begin any of it.

Before my own realization of it, Pennington's high-fat theory had gained some attention and some corroboration elsewhere. Perhaps the most conclusive of the tests to which it was put occurred in Wilmington, Delaware, where the Du Pont company, tried out Pennington's ideas. The subjects were corpulent Du Pont executives who wanted to reduce in order to raise the general level of their health and to achieve maximum efficiency at their jobs.

All the executives involved volunteered, reasoning that they had nothing to lose but weight. The test diet consisted mostly of animal fats, principally sirloin steaks and roasts, so most of the volunteers were actually enthusias-

tic. In most cases, the experiments were entirely successful. The executives lost weight, became ill less frequently
and were reported to be working with higher efficiency.

Another large corporation, Lever Brothers of Cincin-
nati, tried a somewhat similar test. The Lever test diet
stressed vegetable fats rather than animal fats, and 122
students at the Texas State College for Women were the
volunteer subjects. Their aims were improved health,
slimmer figures and better complexions. The tests on the
coeds were conducted by Dr. Pauline Berry Mack, a
prominent nutritionist, and Dr. Mack divided the subjects
into three groups. One group was fed a low-fat diet, another a moderate-fat diet, the third a high-fat diet.

Effectiveness of the experiment varied almost exactly
with the amount of fat consumed. That is, the girls who
ate a moderate-fat diet lost some weight and improved
their complexions somewhat. The girls who ate the high-
fat diet lost more weight and improved their complexions most notably. The girls on a low-fat program fared
poorly. What constituted a high-fat diet to Dr. Mack? One
in which a third of the total caloric intake was composed
of fat.

Lever Brothers had a definite commercial aim in spon-
soring tests of vegetable fats, for the company is a large
producer of vegetable oils and margarine. As a result,
medical and nutritional authorities were somewhat
skeptical about the entire study. This attitude was unfortunate, for, commercial or not, the tests on the Texas
coeds demonstrated a significant point: Vegetable fat was

just as effective as animal fat for a reducing program. This was a fact which some may previously have suspected, but which none previously had proved. It is a fact which was most important to me as I worked out my new nutrition principle. For I was to learn that vegetable and marine fats were *more* important than animal fats.

At roughly the time when the Lever Brothers work was in progress, an article in *Holiday* magazine focused a good deal of public attention on high-fat diets. The article was titled "The Eat-All-You-Want Reducing Diet" and was based on the work of Doctors Donaldson and Pennington. Roughly, it suggested that dieters make 20 per cent of their food lean meat and some 50 per cent of their food fat. In addition, dieters were allowed to eat potatoes and other vegetables low in carbohydrates. Since the article was on the right track, and possibly since the title was catchy, it enjoyed a great deal of success. In 1951 *Holiday* published what might be called a sequel. The magazine now called a high-fat program "The *Holiday* Diet" and offered a program loosely based on the Eskimo diet of Stefansson, the Blake Donaldson diet, the Pennington diet and the Du Pont diet.

For all their prominence, the *Holiday* articles failed to knock out the old low-calorie theories. These lingered, as they still do. But the *Holiday* articles were important as the first prominent national publicity the high-fat principle had received. They also represent a fine example of the progress of medical research. Dr. Donaldson had tried the high-fat principle, discovering that it worked, but not discovering why. Dr. Pennington, who had heard of Dr. Donaldson's work in 1944, applied the principle to himself with marked success and then to a number of others. The work of both men went into the articles.

Dr. Pennington advanced Dr. Donaldson's work with his understanding of what was happening within the human body: namely, the carbohydrate breakdown that I mentioned earlier. He continued to study body chemistry until, tragically, he lost his life in an automobile accident late in 1959.

Recently I have carried the work beyond where Dr. Pennington was forced to leave it. You remember that all calories are not the same, that a calorie of carbohydrate presents a different problem to the body than does a calorie of fat. It is now clear to me that all *fats* are not the same, that there are definite and important differences in the fats you eat. There are differences between animal fats and fish fats and vegetable fats. There are differences, too, in the fats in your blood stream, which are the results of what you eat. There are even differences between the various fat tissues that people want to lose. As we come to understand these differences, we will be closer to an understanding of the new nutrition principle.

# CHAPTER THREE

# WHY SHOULD I
# REDUCE?

ONE CONSIDERATION PRECEDES ALL OTHERS if
any reducing program is to work: You have to want to
reduce. This, may I add, is not as obvious as it sounds.
I am not concerning myself with psychological problems here. I have in mind one important condition: Anyone who wants to reduce must feel strongly enough
about it so that he will adhere to a reasonable reducing
regimen—and adhere to it full time. One cannot follow it
five days a week and hope for results. As you will see, my
principle enforces certain adjustments in eating habits.
Nothing nearly so drastic as the diets you know. Perhaps
substituting cheese for chocolate ice cream as a snack.
Still, you will have to make these readjustments rigidly,
and in this chapter I want to help build your will power.
I want you to see, as I have seen, that fat is not just a
glamour girl's problem. It is a major health problem to
millions and millions of people in every area of life.

I remember frequent drenching rains in Chile. If I went
out and my raincoat leaked, I could raise a justifiable fuss

# MEN

| Height | Age 15–16 | 17–19 | 20–24 | 25–29 | 30–39 | 40–49 | 50–59 | 60–69 |
|---|---|---|---|---|---|---|---|---|
| 5' 0" | 98 | 113 | 122 | 128 | 131 | 134 | 136 | 133 |
| 1" | 102 | 116 | 125 | 131 | 134 | 137 | 139 | 136 |
| 2" | 107 | 119 | 128 | 134 | 137 | 140 | 142 | 139 |
| 3" | 112 | 123 | 132 | 138 | 141 | 144 | 145 | 142 |
| 4" | 117 | 127 | 136 | 141 | 145 | 148 | 149 | 146 |
| 5" | 122 | 131 | 139 | 144 | 149 | 152 | 153 | 150 |
| 6" | 127 | 135 | 142 | 148 | 153 | 156 | 157 | 154 |
| 7" | 132 | 139 | 145 | 151 | 157 | 161 | 162 | 159 |
| 8" | 137 | 143 | 149 | 155 | 161 | 165 | 166 | 163 |
| 9" | 142 | 147 | 153 | 159 | 165 | 169 | 170 | 168 |
| 10" | 146 | 151 | 157 | 163 | 170 | 174 | 175 | 173 |
| 11" | 150 | 155 | 161 | 167 | 174 | 178 | 180 | 178 |
| 6' 0" | 154 | 160 | 166 | 172 | 179 | 183 | 185 | 183 |
| 1" | 159 | 164 | 170 | 177 | 183 | 187 | 189 | 188 |
| 2" | 164 | 168 | 174 | 182 | 188 | 192 | 194 | 193 |
| 3" | 169 | 172 | 178 | 186 | 193 | 197 | 199 | 198 |
| 4" | * | 176 | 181 | 190 | 199 | 203 | 205 | 204 |

# WOMEN

| Height | Age 15–16 | 17–19 | 20–24 | 25–29 | 30–39 | 40–49 | 50–59 | 60–69 |
|---|---|---|---|---|---|---|---|---|
| 4' 10" | 97 | 99 | 102 | 107 | 115 | 122 | 125 | 127 |
| 11" | 100 | 102 | 105 | 110 | 117 | 124 | 127 | 129 |
| 5' 0" | 103 | 105 | 108 | 113 | 120 | 127 | 130 | 131 |
| 1" | 107 | 109 | 112 | 116 | 123 | 130 | 133 | 134 |
| 2" | 111 | 113 | 115 | 119 | 126 | 133 | 136 | 137 |
| 3" | 114 | 116 | 118 | 122 | 129 | 136 | 140 | 141 |
| 4" | 117 | 120 | 121 | 125 | 132 | 140 | 144 | 145 |
| 5" | 121 | 124 | 125 | 129 | 135 | 143 | 148 | 149 |
| 6" | 125 | 127 | 129 | 133 | 139 | 147 | 152 | 153 |
| 7" | 128 | 130 | 132 | 136 | 142 | 151 | 156 | 157 |
| 8" | 132 | 134 | 136 | 140 | 146 | 155 | 160 | 161 |
| 9" | 136 | 138 | 140 | 144 | 150 | 159 | 164 | 165 |
| 10" | * | 142 | 144 | 148 | 154 | 164 | 169 | * |
| 11" | * | 147 | 149 | 153 | 159 | 169 | 174 | * |
| 6' 0" | * | 152 | 154 | 158 | 164 | 174 | 180 | * |

* Average weights omitted in classes having too few cases.

with the man who sold it to me. But he could not stop it from raining.

I can show you a way in which you can reduce, improve your complexion and probably increase your life expectancy. But I cannot stop you from cheating. What I intend to do now is make clear why you should lose the extra weight you are carrying.

Are you carrying extra weight? If you are, how much? For an answer, you had best consult the following table, prepared, after extensive research, by experts at the Metropolitan Life Insurance Company. You should, of course, make allowances for your body build. A small-boned woman of thirty-five who stands 5 feet 5 inches may properly weigh 130 pounds, while a large-boned woman of the same height and age could just as properly weigh 140. But be careful about making such allowances. If you give yourself the benefit of the doubt, you may be giving yourself no benefit at all. You cannot fool your body. You cannot outsmart the life-expectancy figures, which are based to some extent upon these tables.

Here, then, are the averages. Study them and yourself honestly and you will know whether you are carrying extra weight and, if you are, how much extra weight you should lose.

Very technically, there is a distinction between overweight and obesity. A person is said to be overweight if he is five per cent over the established norms. On the other hand obesity, in medical usage, refers to the relationship of body fat to total body weight; when it exceeds eleven per cent, he is obese. In a medical journal or other technical publication, it might be necessary to draw a line between these two terms and use them separately so that the minor distinction would remain clear. But in practice, when a man is overweight, virtually without exception, he is obese. We can use the terms interchangeably except when it is important to distinguish between weight and measurements in inches.

To determine if you are overweight, you simply need step on a scale. Logically if you are more than a pound or two overweight and have neither prodigious muscle nor bone structure, you can assume that you are obese. But there are more precise means of measuring obesity. Take a tape measure and measure first your chest and then your waist. (In women the chest is measured beneath the breasts.) The circumference of your chest should be at least six to eight inches greater than that of your waist. If it is not, you are obese. You are carrying too much extra fat.

Can you gather handfuls of fat by pinching yourself? Is there a visible spare tire of flesh at your waist? Does your abdomen balloon? Do your buttocks protrude? Does your neck pour over your collar? Collectively, these are signs that indicate obesity.

My general rule is that a scale measures overweight and a tape measure measures obesity. Fat is not as compact as muscle. It bulges. A tape measure, or even a sensible look at your body, can tell you whether you are obese.

If after measuring and looking and grabbing for fat,

45

you find that you *are* obese, remember that you're hardly alone. Americans, by and large, are growing more and more obese every year.

Some 20 per cent of all adults in the United States are obese. Not merely by an inch or two, either. They are obese to an extent that impairs their health and their happiness and that has serious and sometimes fatal results. The list of ailments that medical research indicates are worsened or caused by obesity reads like a *Who's Who* of infirmities. It includes heart disease, diabetes, hardening of the arteries, high blood pressure, liver and gall bladder troubles, and disturbances of those key glands called endocrines which secrete vital substances into the blood stream. There is even some evidence that some of the conditions which create obesity have a hand in the growth of cancers.

These are purely physical ills. In addition, there is absolute statistical evidence that obese people are more likely to have accidents. Excess fat does body co-ordination no good; it gives the muscles an extra load to carry. So a fat person is more apt to fall, and when a fat person falls it is considerably more jolting than when a thin person falls— both to the person and to the surroundings.

Finally, there are the emotional disturbances of obesity. The most dramatic evidence here is that fat people are more inclined to suicide than are thin people. This is an abstract statistical fact. Into my office regularly have come unhappy obese women—housewives, professional women, office workers—whose problems were not abstractions; they were as real as the tears these women shed.

There's one pattern I've seen hundreds of times. A man marries a woman because, among other things, he likes her figure. Then, perhaps during pregnancy, perhaps gradually, she puts on a great deal of fat that she is unable to lose. The man looks at his wife one evening and sees, not the figure he had liked, but a figure that strikes him as a caricature. Where there were once curves, there is now flab. Where there was once delicacy, there is now grossness. What was graceful has become plodding. The results of such circumstances are not pleasant for either husband or wife. I have treated numerous obese women whose husbands had stopped having sexual relations with them, apparently because of their obesity. I do not think I am overstating when I say that this is a marital tragedy.

For every woman whose obesity has cost her a normal sex life there are dozens whose obesity has cost them comfort at home. The husband, angry at his wife's weight, convinced that it is her fault, attacks her for a variety of things: her weight, of course, but more than that her dress, her posture, her ability as a homemaker and as a mother. These husbands are distressed, and distress is not always rational.

Besides, many of my patients have admitted to me that when their weight was high they were simply too weary to do a day's housework. They needed more than normal amounts of sleep, they always felt tired, and as a result their homes became messier and messier. An obese woman in a messy house is not the average man's ideal of marriage.

Beyond this, there was a frequent sense of shame. Al-

47

though it was not the fault of anything but medical ignorance and metabolism that these women were fat, many of them were acutely embarrassed. They had, after all, been consulting physicians for many years. They had been given pills 'or injections. They had tried to follow low-calorie diets. "But nothing worked, Doctor," is a phrase I have heard so often that it rings like a refrain. What could these women do—say that a variety of physicians and medical theories had been wrong (which was the case) or decide, privately, that somehow they were wrong, that something they were doing or were not doing was inflicting upon them the despised fat? Most of these women, giving the medical profession the credit it deserves in most areas, could only blame themselves.

Social life often was unwelcome. Who wants to be stared at or whispered about? (Sometimes an obese person thinks others are staring and whispering even when they are not.) Shopping for clothes was close to agony. Black hides fat, so obese people favor it, but the prospect of buying a tent-sized dress from a slim salesgirl gave many of my patients painful moments. The swimming season was sheer horror. Few obese people like the idea of squeezing into a bathing suit, but, come summer, many obese people are led off to beaches by their children. The beach should be a place of enjoyment. But it is not if you bring with you pounds and pounds of extra fat. After I have introduced you to the new nutrition principle, I will introduce you to some case histories. Many of them include proud statements like "And now I can go to the beach."

An outstanding source of life-expectancy charts in the United States is the vast Metropolitan Life Insurance Company. It is this company's business to estimate how long someone will live before selling him a life insurance policy, because, of course, premium rates are based on the number of years the policy buyer has left. The better the estimates, the more efficiently this company can operate. So its studies have been exhaustive.

According to recent research by the company, the death rate for obese men ranged up to 75 per cent higher than that for men of normal weight. For obese women the rate was as much as 61 per cent above normal. Moderately obese men and women had a death rate roughly 50 per cent above the national average.

Let's break this down a little further. People 15 or 20 pounds overweight—almost invariably obese—have a death rate 10 per cent higher than normal. The rate grows proportionately higher with the poundage—at an average of one year per pound! So every extra pound you put on increases your chance of dying before your time. If you are 85 pounds overweight, you have an 85 per cent greater chance of dying early than does a person of normal weight. Consider these figures carefully, and then consider your own figure. There is more than glamour involved in keeping slim. It can be a matter of life and death.

Many reputable American insurance companies turn down thousands of obese applicants every year. Why? Because records prove that fat people are bad insurance risks. Dead weight is clearly a term that can be literal.

Even when an insurance company accepts an obese applicant, he is often required to pay an extra premium. Most of the obese people who die before their time are killed by diabetes, diseases of the digestive tract or heart disease. One Metropolitan Life Insurance study of ailments that are usually serious and sometimes fatal showed this:

The incidence of cerebral hemorrhage—hemorrhage within the brain, something which can kill or paralyze victims—runs 60 per cent higher among the overweight.

The incidence of chronic nephritis—inflammation of the kidneys, something which can lead to an agonizing death—runs 90 per cent higher among the overweight.

There are four times as many overweight diabetics as diabetics of normal weight. Three times as many overweight people suffer from cirrhosis of the liver, often fatal, as do normal people. Of course, this liver condition may be associated with alcoholism, and alcoholism may be associated with extra poundage. But even among non-alcoholics, cirrhosis is far more common in the fat than in the slim. Let's take a longer look at some of the chronic diseases influenced or brought on by overweight (enough extra poundage so that we can presume obesity):

*Cancer.* As you know, cancer remains a medical mystery. Certain studies, for example, indicate that irritation contributes to cancerous conditions in some. But not in all. Irritation alone cannot be said to cause cancer. Nor can any other single factor. This is a highly complex condition—unfortunately, more complex than modern medicine has been able to learn. But of obesity and cancer we do know this: Extra poundage appears to make people more prone to death from the disease. The cancer death rate is 10 per cent higher among the obese than it is among the normal. Insurance company figures reveal, further, that among all the men who bought policies at forty-five or older, those whose weight was 15 per cent or more above normal had a cancer death rate fully 25 per cent higher than those of average weight. So if you are over forty-five and are overweight, you are increasing a chance you'd just as soon cut down: your chance of being stricken by cancer. There is other research that indicates obese women have a 30 to 45 per cent greater chance of developing cancer of the uterus than do normal women.

Again, let me make clear, neither I nor any other responsible medical researcher would assert that obesity by itself causes cancer. But the statistical evidence is there for all to see. And when considering something as serious as cancer, does it make sense to argue with statistics? I think not, and I'm certain you agree.

Some interesting research has been undertaken in England to establish, if possible, a relationship between diet and cancer. In short, by eating the traditional diet, rich in carbohydrates, are we creating a body climate which is conducive to the growth of cancers? Some results have been published which indicate that certain vegetable fats inhibit the growth of cancer in laboratory animals. Animals are not humans, and this line of research is only at its beginning. But the considerable statistical evidence we have correlates obesity with cancer, and the frac-

51

tional amount of experimental evidence we have indicates that there may be some hope for combating cancer through diet, perhaps only as one of several ways of battling this killer. This is worthy of serious consideration. Your own physician should be able to inform you on further investigations into the relationship between cancer and diet.

*Heart Disease.* Like cancer, this remains a mystery and, as such, remains a killer. But here the evidence against fat is far more conclusive. Consider this one point: Obese persons with heart disease—that is, those who have a chronic condition or who have already had at least one coronary seizure—have a death rate 44 per cent higher than do normal people who have had heart attacks. It is no mystery that excess poundage puts an added strain on anyone's heart. But it is not as well known that there is a growing body of medical evidence that heart attacks are not caused by blood clots, the belief of former days. This evidence has led many doctors to conclude that the cause of heart attacks will be discovered in the blood vessels. What does fat do to the blood vessels? This leads us to consider the disease called arteriosclerosis, or hardening of the arteries.

*Diseases of Veins and Arteries.* A recent survey was made of 22,741 officers in the United States Army, both men and women, on the effects of weight. It showed that among both men and women of every age blood pressure increased steadily in proportion to body weight. Hypertension, the medical term for high blood pressure, develops in overweight people two and a half times as often as it does in people of normal weight. Even more startling were results of a study conducted by the American Society of Actuaries (the men who work out life-expectancy tables). This showed that even a relatively small increase in weight lifted blood pressure perceptibly and that small increases in blood pressure increased death rates to a greater degree than anyone had suspected.

What all this means is clear to physicians and should be clear to you. Heart disease is our number one killer and we can be certain that both high blood pressure and hardening of the arteries make things more difficult for the heart. Why do fat people have higher blood pressure? Probably because the extra fat puts a special burden on the circulatory system; there is more tissue for the blood to reach. Why do fat people suffer more from hardening of the arteries, sometimes developing arteries that are hard as stone? No one is quite sure of the reason, but we are sure that a relationship between this disease and obesity exists.

I cannot stress too strongly that, in the entire area of heart and blood-vessel diseases, we are dealing with life —yours, mine and our children's. Over one third of all Americans alive now will die of diseases associated with hardening of the arteries, according to the best estimates. Thin people don't live forever, but their chances of premature hardening of the arteries, of the painful and unpleasant conditions that go hand in hand with this killer, are notably lessened. If you are heavy now and you lose weight, the chances of your death from hardening of the arteries will be considerably lessened. Even if you have been fat for years, it is not too late.

*Diabetes.* This disease, in its most common form, is marked by the body's inability to use sugar properly. What does this mean? At its mildest, sugar in the urine; at its most severe, instant death.

You may have heard diabetes described as "fat man's folly." Almost eight out of ten diabetic persons are obese when symptoms first appear. There are responsible medical estimates that weight reduction alone could prevent a substantial number of the diabetes cases in America. Approximately two million Americans are victims at present.

Women are more prone to obesity than men, and women are more prone to diabetes. In Holland recently there was research that clearly demonstrated that excess fat, and not a sexual predisposition, explained the greater number of diabetic women. At the same time, it demonstrated that insulin, which burns sugar and is the standard treatment for diabetics, is not in itself enough. Proper diet —low carbohydrate intake—is essential, too.

I've seen further research which shows that only one person in twenty is underweight when diabetic symptoms appear and that among people who are forty or over, nine out of ten who come down with diabetes are overweight. "Fat man's folly" is a reasonable name. Again the thin are more likely to skip the hardships of a grave disease.

*Hernia.* This condition, which is most common in men

and is sometimes referred to as a "rupture," may be partly caused by excess weight.

In hernia a body canal, usually in the abdomen, breaks through a wall of tissue that keeps it in place. This, of course, can be quite painful. The protruding tissue is called the sac, and at one time physicians believed that a diet that reduced the size of the sac might be dangerous. Generally, they were concerned about changing the make-up of the sac. If it was heavily fat, let it remain that way, they believed. But recently it has been learned that general fat reduction, including reduction of the size of the sac, improves a hernia condition. This seems to indicate that fat contributes to a hernia; certainly it doesn't help the condition.

*Gynecological and Obstetrical Complications.* A normally proportioned woman is more likely to give birth to a healthy baby than is a woman who is obese. She is more likely to have a safe and comfortable pregnancy and far less likely to be stricken with toxemia, the body poisoning which is so serious in pregnant women. When she is not pregnant, the normally proportioned woman is less likely to suffer from menstrual difficulties. She is more likely to conceive children.

*Other Effects.* Not all of the results of obesity are as grave as heart disease, as troubling as infertility. Some are merely annoying. Aching feet are hardly likely to prove fatal, but they are something less than enjoyable. Foot troubles are particularly prevalent among the obese. So are heat rashes, pains in the joints, sleeplessness and different types of incorrect posture. Carrying extra weight is a strain, affecting every part of the body.

One condition which is usually no more than annoying can, under certain conditions, become serious. It is impeded respiration brought on by fat. Because the body has to do more work to move and because it is burdened with so much extra tissue, the fat person often is short of breath. Ordinarily this is annoying or embarrassing; in an operating room it represents another problem. Most deep anesthesia involves the inhalation of a gas, and for normal people this anesthesia is quite safe. But for someone who is obese, anesthesia can be a risky business. An obese person's breathing mechanism is always under strain. Anesthesia increases the strain, and there have been cases in which the extra strain has proved fatal.

Many hospitals are now reluctant to perform certain types of surgery on the obese. The surgeon's job is more difficult if he must cut through thick layers of fat, but the real problem is the anesthetist's. If respiratory anesthesia is necessary, some anesthetists take the flat stand that the risk on an obese person is too great to justify the surgery. So here is a minor complication of obesity, shortness of breath, which can become a major complication at a time when the obese person is facing surgery and probably has enough complications already.

*Psychological Aspects.* A common and somber psychological problem is this: An emotional disturbance starts a person on the way to obesity. Then, in frantic, futile attempts to reduce, the person worsens the original emotional problem. It would be difficult to imagine a more vicious circle.

Generally speaking, there are two types of obesity which seem to be psychologically caused. One type is called, simply, psychological obesity; the other is developmental obesity.

Psychological obesity usually starts in middle age after some particularly disturbing experience. It may be a serious operation; it may be prolonged illness, the death of a friend or the end of a love affair. It may even be a business crisis or homesickness. The disturbed person then begins to eat as an escape, as something to do. Almost invariably he concentrates on carbohydrates—candy, ice cream, cake. The search for a release fails and creates instead the additional emotional crisis of obesity.

Developmental obesity, the common childhood type, involves the whole personality. A child who is insecure, anxious, unsuccessful, finds a refuge in overeating. He shuns ordinary social contacts and activities for deep-seated psychological reasons, but, as his overeating transforms his appearance, he blames the extra weight. "Nobody likes me because I'm fat," he may say, ignoring the fact that he wasn't liked a few years earlier when he was slim. He has confused the symptom with the cause.

The Iowa Agricultural and Home Economics Experiment Stations in Ames have made personality studies on a sampling of rural girls who were severely overweight. The studies have shown consistent patterns of emotional disturbance, correlated with the fat. As against the average, obese girls did less well in school and had less understanding and acceptance of sex. Their relationships with their parents, particularly their mothers, were precarious. Finally, they were physically less active.

Just what is cause and what is effect would vary with each individual case. Generalizations about psychology are dangerous. But there is one that I am convinced is right. Obese people, on the basis of all the evidence we have, are less happy than people of normal weight.

There is one final, curious point about psychological obesity. Many of my patients always ate fattening foods at certain times and under certain conditions. One woman ate chocolate ice cream whenever she watched television. She watched TV every night, as her figure showed. Others eat while playing cards, while listening to music, while relaxing. It is as if these people cannot follow the theme of a symphony or the plot of a television Western without the aid of a large platter of ice cream. Usually, after I called their attention to it these people were able to break the pattern in a few months. Sometimes they broke it easily, but in several cases they succeeded only by barring ice cream from their homes.

"We had guests the other night," one of these women told me, "and I served them ice cream. But as soon as they left, I took all the ice cream that was left and threw it out." Then, for a snack, she ate a few sardines, which, as marine fat and protein, were fine.

By and large, this chapter has been a bit somber, but if you are obese and the chapter has awakened you to a need for action, then it has served its purpose. It has not been my aim to frighten you into acting, but only to make you aware so that you can take steps rationally. For our whole current problem of obesity can be examined rationally, just as it can be conquered rationally.

Why is extra fat so grave a problem now? Well, fifty years ago only 62 per cent of the babies born were expected to reach the age of forty-five. Today that figure has risen to 90 per cent. Victories over the infectious diseases are what have raised the figure and have given so many of us so many more years of life. It is all-important to make these extra years healthful ones, for there is an ever increasing proportion of Americans who are in the middle or the late time of life.

Medical science gives us the extra years. Are we going to let obesity and its hazards rob us of the advantages these years can bring? Not if everyone understands the seriousness of putting on excess weight at any time in life. Not if everyone recognizes obesity as the killer and crippler that it is. Not if everyone accepts the fact that, just as we conquered smallpox and pneumonia, we must now move ahead to conquer obesity.

# CHAPTER FOUR

# FOOD, FADS AND
# FALLACIES

ALTHOUGH OBESITY HAS BECOME an increasing problem as man's life span has lengthened, it did not suddenly become so with the advent of modern medicine. Obesity is as old as civilization. And, as you may remember from my comments on agricultural and hunters' diets, it is civilization itself that we must blame for the creation of obesity. Man, building a more comfortable life, has also built himself a more expansive paunch.

As far as we can tell, obesity was almost unknown among the prehistoric races. It is still rare among the surviving primitives, such as the Veddas of Ceylon and the aborigines of Australia. The life expectancy of primitive man was eighteen years; anyone surviving to the age of forty was a patriarch. The primitives lived violent lives and frequently died violent deaths. Then, with the coming of civilization, its comfort, its calm, its agriculture, there followed obesity.

Evidence is clear in writings from early civilizations. There is the Bible story of Israel, who gorged himself on fats and sweets, grew waxy, pale and so enormously obese that he was "disgusting before the Lord." The Talmud, an ancient Hebrew commentary, tells of a rabbi who grew so obese that his belly was opened and "baskets of fat were removed."

In general, the rule seems to be that the more highly developed the civilization, the greater the incidence of obesity. Both the diet of civilization, overly rich in carbohydrates, and the role of age in obesity contribute toward this rule.

Even among such highly developed races as the ancient Greeks, the average life expectancy was only thirty years. Only nine Greeks out of a hundred lived to be sixty-eight, which is the average life span of the slender American today.

Why is age so significant to obesity? As one grows older, tissues deteriorate, and when muscle tissue deteriorates it is usually replaced by fat. Perhaps if all of us lived more actively this deterioration would be slowed. But the older we get, the less exercise we are likely to take. The shipping clerk who loaded packages becomes a section manager and sits behind a desk. The policeman who walked a beat becomes a sergeant and rides in a patrol car. The bank messenger who scooted about becomes a personal loan consultant, and people come to him. The active young mother becomes less active as her children grow older and require less by way of frantic pursuit. If her husband is successful, she may acquire a maid. This frees her from the chore of housework, which as any woman can testify is exercise of a sort. All too frequently she devotes most of her new leisure to such sedentary activities as bridge.

Athletes provide a most dramatic illustration of the sedentary aging. Many athletes are overweight when judged against the tables of average weight. This is not to say the athletes are obese. Their heavy muscle structure makes them weigh more than other men of the same size. Training keeps the athlete's muscle structure heavy, so when you read that a six-foot football lineman weighs 225 pounds, you can reasonably assume that what he's carrying is extra muscle, not extra blubber. All well and good.

Then the athlete reaches an age when he can no longer stand the rigors of competition. Sometimes his skills fade gradually; sometimes they disappear with startling abruptness. Now the heavy-muscled athlete, who is perhaps thirty-five years old, must embark on another career. Whatever he chooses, wherever he is accepted, the new career will not utilize all those muscles that have been built up so painfully for so long. The athlete, who once ran for several hours a day, now sits behind a desk. The muscles, which may be starting to deteriorate slightly anyway—why else would his active career have ended?— deteriorate with extra speed because they are no longer being utilized.

A year after he has stopped playing football, that six-foot lineman may still weigh 225 pounds. But now he is more than overweight. He is obese. He has lost muscle and added fat. The hard muscular lines of his ample frame have softened. He has a bulge behind his neck and another at the middle. This, mind you, if he holds his weight. If he adds weight, then his problem is compounded; he too may become "disgusting before the Lord."

To a good many people of middle years, life is a constant battle of the bulge. Now with proper dietary habits and a reasonable amount of exercise, the battle need never be fought. But in the years when physicians were unable to define "proper dietary habits," food fads and starvation diets became part of our national pattern. They were parlor games, so to speak, in which everyone played to lose. In the light of current medical knowledge, it is clear that these fads and diets did far more harm than good.

Fat women—and remember, the majority of obese people are women—are easy prey to all sorts of fads and fallacies. Most women, out of consideration for their health, their husbands or their illusions, would rather not weigh too much, and with all the best intentions they become victims of strange diets and "beauty culture" businesses which thrive on massage, calisthenics, dancing, exercise and nonsense. These women make a great many people rich, not only people who invent odd diets or formulate techniques of beauty culture, but responsible businessmen as well. In an average year, American women purchase 640 million dollars' worth of girdles and 2.5 million dollars' worth of bathroom scales. That represents a lot of girdling and a lot of weighing.

As we have seen, low-calorie diets are without scientific basis, but calorie-consciousness has paid off handsomely for many commercial companies. More than two hundred firms produce what they advertise as "low-calorie" foods, and they produce them by the carload. The best estimate is that a quarter of a billion dollars' worth of low-calorie food is sold in the United States each year. The low-calorie soft drink is a comparative newcomer. In 1952 fifty thousand cases were sold. By 1958 the figure had leaped to fifteen million. And it is still increasing. (Since the calories in soft drinks were carbohydrate, these new drinks actually are an improvement.)

Once more, let me emphasize the dangers in embarking on a crash diet. Starve yourself and you greatly increase your chances of developing a serious condition called ptosis. In ptosis, abdominal walls collapse, leaving unsupported such vital organs as the kidneys and the intestines.

Dr. Frederick J. Stare, who is the director of the department of nutrition at Harvard, summarizes the perils of crash dieting extremely well:

There is no more cure for overweight than insulin for diabetes. (Insulin, of course, is a treatment, not a cure.) At best, diets enable you to control your illness. At worst, as in fad dieting, they trap you in a vicious circle of losing and gaining, which is not only futile but, quite possibly, dangerous. Among illnesses that may possibly be precipitated by off-again, on-again crash dieting are rheumatic fever and asthma, high blood pressure, arteriosclerosis, gout, thyroid disease and others. One New York faddist was even hospitalized for scurvy—the only such case the doctors had seen in fifty years.

Mankind seems to have a natural weakness for food fads, whether to control fat or for other reasons. The religions of the world are filled with dietary laws, often written without scientific basis. The great Pythagoras surrendered to pursuing enemies in 500 B.C. when the enemies had driven him to the edge of a bean field. Beans, he believed, were contaminating and he chose death as preferable to contamination. There is an equal amount of reason in some of the fads of today. Let's consider a few:

*Drugs and Elixirs.* The old-time medicine man could cure anything, including obesity. "Step right up," he barked, "and, for just a little silver, purchase this bottle of Smith's Patented Cure-All, good for stiff joints, catarrh and— What's that, madam, will it get rid of your fat? It'll melt it, like the sunshine melts the snow! Twenty-five cents, please."

Today's reducing drugs are advertised with a greater degree of subtlety, but all seem to proceed from the principle that the end—weight loss—justifies any means. The label on the bottle will list what the drug contains, usually in terms that are meaningless to laymen, but it is a rare label that admits that the contents can produce a wide variety of side effects.

Many slimming medicines use a thyroid extract as a base. If you have a marked thyroid deficiency, the extract

67

may help you, but its effect on general obesity is questionable. There is simply no scientific evidence that thyroid extract will help cure obesity unless the obesity is caused by thyroid defect. Only a physician is qualified to measure the condition of a thyroid gland.

Now suppose a thyroid extract makes your fat disappear, can you then assume that a thyroid defect is causing your obesity? Even here you cannot be sure. The complete function of the thyroid gland is not fully understood. So perhaps the extract is helping your thyroid or perhaps it is working through a process which even physicians do not comprehend. You are playing with unknowns, a dangerous sport. We do know that thyroid extract can elevate blood pressure and can worsen a heart condition. I would say that if you suffer from any circulatory disease, or from diabetes, and you take thyroid extract pills without consulting a physician, you actually are endangering your life.

Iodine is another element widely used in slimming drugs, and there is no question but that certain quantities of iodine are essential to the human system. But taking iodine on your own, taking it in unspecified doses, is something else. Too much iodine has woeful effects on the skin. Rashes and pimples and deep-rooted skin diseases are some of the side effects.

Other drugs, sheer fakes, are nothing more than laxatives. Of course eliminating bulk reduces weight—until your next meal. It's like the steam cabinet that reduces weight until the next drink of water. Neither a laxative nor a product that induces frequent urination has any real effect on the fat you want to lose.

Many of the drugs and elixirs offer a reducing plan or formula to go along with them. Bear in mind that the claims made for most of these drugs are absurd. The plans and formulas are usually just as irrational.

My own advice is a reminder that drugs taken without medical advice are dangerous, and that as yet there is no valid drug or medicine that can make you lose weight naturally and—just as important—keep you at the proper weight level. There is not a single patent medicine being marketed now that I would recommend to a patient as a means of weight control.

The popularity of commercial weight-control products is easily measured. How popular, then, are home remedies? Obviously, they too must be widely followed, but, since obesity remains a problem, they cannot be very effective. Here are some home cures for extra weight:

*Lemon Juice.* According to the formula of many grandmothers, lemon juice will help you lose weight. The grandmothers can't tell you why they believe this; possibly because they heard it from their own grandmothers years before. The scientific evidence is that the vitamin C in lemon juice helps repair worn-out tissue but does not destroy fat. Nor does the citric acid that lemon juice contains. Lemon juice may be healthful as a source of nutrients, but it is valueless as a treatment for obesity.

*A Morning Glass of Water.* Many people believe that a glass of water on arising is a sure cure for excess poundage. Why? Water won't dissolve away fat—fat does not dissolve in water. For some, of course, there is a psychological effect. After all, people reason, sugar pills have cured many ailments; can't water, then, cure obesity? Unfortunately it cannot, whether taken at arising, on retiring, or in between. Proper intake of water is important in a general reducing program, as we shall see later, but by itself the water has no value other than the fact that it fills your stomach. Filling the stomach with water instead of carbohydrates may have some effect on weight, but obviously the total effect will be small. Water is not a substitute for food.

*Toast Instead of Bread.* A common fallacy holds that toast is less fattening than bread. Another holds that the crust of bread is less fattening than the softer portions. As I say, these are fallacies. Both are erroneous, each in its way.

When you toast a piece of bread, you are removing water from it. Nothing else. Only water. If you eat as much toast as you would eat bread, the relative amount of carbohydrate you consume is actually higher. This is one reason why toast is recommended to people who are recovering from illness and should gain weight. Diets which advocate "one piece of dry toast" are unsound. One piece of dry bread would be better, although if you are seriously overweight neither is really good for you. Bread is a high-carbohydrate food, and whether it is whole-wheat bread, rye bread, white bread or the commercially advertised "protein bread" this is still true.

70

The crust actually contains more concentrated carbohydrate than any other portion of the bread. The same principle that applies to toast applies here as well. Bread acquires a crust as it is baked; the crust is the portion from which the most water has been removed. Just as a diet urging toast is senseless, someone urging you to concentrate on bread crusts is being illogical, too. In almost any form, bread is fattening.

*Dried Fruits Instead of Fresh Fruits.* Once more we are dealing with the fallacious notion that water makes fat. Yet there are many people who believe that dried fruits are better than fresh fruits for people who want to reduce. These people are totally in error.

The dried fruits are highly concentrated carbohydrate; they are extremely fattening. Figs, dates, raisins, dried apricots and peaches are, in their effect on the obese, nothing more than concentrated fat. Even fresh fruits—notably apples and bananas—have a high carbohydrate concentrate and can have a startling effect on weight gain. Some of Dr. Pennington's patients, treated with his high-fat diet, gained weight when they ate a single apple; sometimes even half an apple was enough, or too much.

It may seem strange to you that so small a quantity of food can cause a weight gain. I know many of my patients wonder if a little fruit will affect them. They always find out, sadly, that it does. For the body of someone with a weight problem seems almost to be waiting for carbohydrates. As soon as a concentration of carbohydrate is eaten, the body chemistry works with remarkable speed to

71

produce fat. Unfortunately, the fat cannot be lost as quickly.

*Whiskey and Water.* There is a misconception here that often stems from wishful thinking: It's the soda, not the Scotch, that's making me fat. But we must face a blunt truth: It's the whiskey, not the soda, that creates the glow —and creates the fat.

Alcohol, a carbohydrate, has a high caloric content. An ounce of whiskey contains 100 carbohydrate calories. Six ounces of cola or a sweet drink, such as ginger ale, contain seventy-five calories of carbohydrate. For a long time people who liked to drink concentrated on eliminating the extra carbohydrate by taking their drinks mixed with water. (Lately, with the development of soft drinks all but free of carbohydrate content, these drinkers have been able to go back to their favorite mixers.) But an ounce of whiskey is an ounce of whiskey, in whatever combination you drink it. And an ounce of whiskey is fattening.

It is my belief that wine with meals serves as an aid to digestion. This is because of the acidity of wine; acid is important to the digestive process. Many European races have been drinking wine with meals over the centuries, both as a digestive aid and because good drinking water was harder to get than was good wine. I don't think a small glass of wine at dinner makes anyone fat, nor is it likely to impede weight loss. But three or four ounces of whiskey a day, with soda, with water or straight, is something else. If you are trying to lose weight, I would suggest that you stop drinking whiskey or limit yourself to one drink a day at the most.

*Skipping Potatoes.* Are potatoes fattening? Not when you compare them to bread, cereal or apples. Carbohydrates form only one fifth of the weight of a potato, and, with identical portions, bread produces twice as many calories of carbohydrate as does a potato.

Why, then, the widespread belief that potatoes make you fat? I can only conclude that the problem is not the potato itself but the way in which the potato is prepared. French-fried potatoes, cooked in lard, are fattening food. Lard—highly concentrated *animal* fat—is the culprit. The same principle applies to potatoes fried in *solid* vegetable fat. Solid vegetable fat undergoes a process called hydrogenation, which makes it extremely fattening. Again, the potato itself is not guilty. The truth is that a potato properly prepared is a valuable adjunct to the correct sort of high-fat diet. I'd like to see the spud regain its rightful place on the table. It belongs there.

*Skipping Soups.* Some soups are fattening; some are not. Marrow fat, an animal fat, is used in preparing many soups, which is, perhaps, the origin of the belief that all soups are fattening. Actually, soups with high carbohydrate content—flour, cereals, lentils—are the ones that I believe are most damaging and the ones to avoid.

*Skipping Lunch.* Millions of American workers either skip lunch entirely or eat a small snack instead of a full meal. For many the reason is economy or time, but for the obese the reason is a hoped-for loss in weight. It will shock most of these obese people to learn that when they skip lunch they may be contributing toward weight *gain*. How can *not* eating make anyone fat? The answer involves a basic body principle called "waste heat," which is really quite simple.

Food has an effect on everyone's metabolism—roughly, the sum of the chemical processes concerned with body growth, repair and maintenance. What food does is raise the metabolic rate. As the metabolic rate rises, this waste heat is produced. It is called waste heat because it cannot be converted into physical energy or stored as fat. All it does is raise the body temperature slightly. Waste heat lasts in the body for six to eight hours, no more.

Now, while this waste heat is in evidence the body is burning fuel, working at a faster rate, but it is not accumulating extra fat. Remember, waste heat cannot be stored as fat. So waste heat is an advantage to the obese. By skipping a lunch and losing the benefit of waste heat, a fat person may end up gaining weight as the body works more slowly on the food already in his system.

The chemistry, perhaps, may be less important to you than the results. And one result of the process of waste heat is this: The body works better on three meals a day than on two or on one. When you divide your food among three meals, your metabolism is elevated for from twelve to eighteen hours out of the twenty-four. When you eat one or two large meals, your metabolism is elevated very briefly; your body stores more fat.

*Semistarvation.* Among the really desperate, starvation is one of the most common techniques of losing weight—

or, more accurately, of trying to lose weight. There are a number of reasons why starvation does not work as a practical treatment. The major one is this: Starvation reduces weight not simply by reducing the amount of fat in the body, but by reducing the amount of all body tissue. As a matter of fact, fat often goes late, long after vital muscle tissue has been consumed by the body in its effort to sustain itself on little or no food.

I caution you strongly against attempting to starve yourself. Starvation is accompanied by weakness, lethargy, constipation and other disturbing side effects. Further, the person trying to starve himself is making no effort to correct the original cause of his excess weight. Success, therefore, can be obtained only by undernourishing the entire body, and it can be maintained only the same way. The long-range consequences of malnutrition are numerous and disastrous.

I am not, of course, suggesting that if you starve yourself you will not lose weight. You will. But not in the way you hoped. And when you stop fasting, as ultimately you must, you may regain more weight than you lost, and if you tend toward obesity you will gain more *fat* than you lost. We can discuss this more fully in the next chapter, which deals with the biggest fallacy of all, the low-calorie diet.

*Low-Sodium Diets.* Salt, chemically, is sodium chloride, so ordinary table salt is a prime source of sodium. A salt-free diet, then, is a low-sodium diet. This regimen has certain merits, but it cannot cure obesity.

How much salt does a normal person need? The answer

depends largely on what he eats. Races which subsist largely on vegetables seem to require a great deal of salt; they hunger for it. So do vegetable-eating tropical animals. A salt lick in the jungle is often crowded with animals, busily devouring salt. On the other hand, Eskimos abhor salt. So do meat-eating animals.

Cereals and certain vegetables contain a good deal of potassium, and we know, from certain studies, that eating foods which are rich in potassium will lower the sodium level in the body. In response to this, the body develops an actual salt hunger to fill its need. Have you felt genuine salt hunger? Probably not, for on the basis of clinical evidence it appears that the average American eats too much salt.

Our diet is rich in sodium. Some meats, particularly ham, bacon, salted pork and the white meat of poultry, and some sea food, particularly lobsters, crabs, mussels and clams, are prime sources of sodium. The individual who eats these foods and, in addition, relishes such things as pickles, sauerkraut, salted crackers and salted nuts, is almost certainly taking in an excess of sodium. Further, present food-processing methods use a number of sodium compounds as preservatives. It is safe for the average American to assume that he needs very little extra salt.

Many physicians prescribe low-sodium diets as treatment for complications that result from obesity or go hand in hand with it. High blood pressure and certain skin conditions are examples. But in these cases, the physician is treating a complication; he is not treating obesity.

It is a mistake to believe that salt will help you gain or lose weight. It does neither significantly.

*Low-Fat Diets.* It is easy to understand how low-fat diets became popular. It was natural to assume that what caused fat was probably fat itself. A natural assumption, but one that, in the light of present knowledge, is incorrect.

Several things happen within your body when you restrict fat intake. The body readily converts carbohydrates into fat—and on a low-fat diet you will probably eat a great deal of carbohydrate-rich food. Then the presence of so much carbohydrate impedes the fat-mobilizing activity of the pituitary gland. What is fat mobilizing? A stage the body undergoes when ridding itself of fat. Further, the extra carbohydrate increases the fat-depositing activity of insulin. What is fat depositing? Exactly what it appears to be: the depositing of fat around the body.

So in almost every possible way a low-fat diet makes you put on more fat. Your body does not get rid of fat at its normal rate; it adds fat at a rate faster than normal, and all the ingredients it needs to make fat are available in carbohydrates. The low-fat diet does exactly the opposite of what it is supposed to do. It makes you gain weight.

There is another significant drawback to a low-fat diet. It's almost always deficient in bulk. Now, bulk is important in controlling appetite. Without bulk you suffer from a more or less constant feeling of emptiness, and you

77

are likely to eat more than you normally would. So on yet one more count the low-fat diet fails.

Finally, the low-fat diet, like most other fads and fallacies, fails to work any significant lasting change in a person's eating habits. Even if such a diet did work, it would not work for long. The weight loser after a time would return to his normal eating pattern.

The golden rule of weight reduction is this: Any method of losing weight must first of all correct the underlying cause of the original weight gain. Unless it does, it cannot be permanently successful.

All of this leads us to the most widely believed fallacy in the American nutritional pattern: the belief that low-calorie diets are an effective means of reducing. This supposition, so erroneous but so widespread, deserves a chapter to itself.

# CHAPTER FIVE

# WHY LOW-CALORIE DIETS DON'T WORK

OUR EATING HABITS ARE slow to form and hard to break. Once they have been developed over decades or over centuries, we tend to cling to them, regardless of logic. A distinguished American physician once suggested quite seriously that if it were proved that some mysterious substance in white bread caused cancer, people would go right on eating white bread for the next twenty years. We do what we are accustomed to doing.

American eating habits are a curious mixture, arrived at over centuries. Immigrants from a variety of lands brought a variety of dietary patterns with them. And, as one physiologist has pointed out, an immigrant will abandon the language of his fatherland before he abandons the eating pattern on which he was brought up.

How difficult is it to change eating habits? During one stage of World War II, the populace of Malta, an island base of the Royal Air Force which was all but cut off by the Luftwaffe, was close to starvation. Constant bombing tore at the island. Ships bound for Malta were bombed or torpedoed. In this emergency, the British distributed emergency foods, such as powdered eggs and powdered milk. Starving Maltese actually threw the powdered food out of their houses into the streets. They weren't used to powdered food; they didn't want it, even when faced with starvation.

From Asia comes a parallel case. During an Indian famine some years ago the rice supply ran out. Relief workers offered the Hindus a cereal grass called millet. There are cases of Hindus who starved to death in preference to switching from rice to millet.

Such incidents are extreme, of course, yet in perspective they help explain the persistent popularity of low-calorie diets. The American bill of fare includes puddings from England, sauces from France, grains and meats from ancient Europe, and turkey, corn and pumpkin from American Indians. It is a heterogeneous diet, as our country itself is heterogeneous. But one aspect of the American diet is unique. That is the almost universal belief that calories create fat.

Ours is not the only country in the world where low-calorie diets are popular. But in no other country is the degree of popularity so great, is the use of low-calorie diets more extensive, is the myth of calorie counting accepted more devoutly.

As we have seen, fact and fantasy are closely intertwined in theories and treatment of obesity. Half-truths survive as facts. Falsehoods survive as half-truths. The old-time snake oil salesman was no less a fraud than are some of today's so-called diet specialists, who recommend fantastic foods and fads to a desperate audience of the obese.

Current belief in low-calorie diets rests on two assumptions:

1. Low-calorie diets are effective.
2. Low-calorie diets are harmless.

According to recent studies which have been published in the American Medical Association's *Archives of Internal Medicine*, a completely, authoritative publication, neither of these assumptions is true.

These were not casual studies. Some of them considered low-calorie diets and people who had tried them as reported in medical literature over a period of thirty years. All the people studied firsthand were outpatients, which is to say they were treated at hospitals while living at home. This is important, because hospitals have superior facilities for whatever tests physicians may want to make in treating obesity.

Among the outpatients, all of whom were grossly overweight, only 25 per cent were able to lose as much as 20 pounds. For someone who is grossly overweight, this is hardly a significant success. Forty pounds might be more like it, but only 5 per cent of the obese outpatients were able to lose forty pounds.

Why, then, do people follow low-calorie diets? Because dietary habits persist, regardless of logic.

A similar study was made on 100 obese people who, for treatment, went to the Nutrition Clinic of the New York Hospital, an outstanding medical institution. Over a three-month period Dr. Mavis McLaren-Hume interviewed every person admitted to the clinic. The general health of the patients was good. Ninety-seven were women; three were men. The average excess weight was 44 pounds, with extremes ranging from 21 to 119 pounds overweight, measured against insurance company tables. The average age of the patients was forty-five. In short, this was a cross section of fat Americans of middle age who wanted urgently to reduce.

Several low-calorie balanced diets were tried on the patients. (Calorie intake varied with the different diets from 800 to 1,500 a day.) The patients were examined at intervals of from two to six weeks and no drugs were used. Clearly, this was a low-calorie program designed for safety as well as for weight reduction.

Two and a half years later the patients were again checked for a final tally. Only twelve of the 100 patients had succeeded in losing more than 20 pounds *at any time* during the two and a half years. Only one of the twelve had ever lost more than 40 pounds. Of the twelve who had lost 20 pounds, half had regained weight within a year after the loss. All but two had regained weight within two years. The rate of success was, then, 2 per cent. That is, only two people out of a hundred who went to an outstanding medical clinic and tried low-calorie diets under the best possible conditions enjoyed any real success. As medical treatment, this is about as effective as what we do for the common cold. We can do nothing for the common cold except wait for it to go away. Under low-calorie diets, we can do almost nothing for obesity. And, unlike a cold, obesity does not go away in a week or ten days. It is a chronic ailment.

Remember, too, that these low-calorie diets were planned with safety in mind. Every effort was made to prevent any unpleasant side effects. Despite this, twenty-one of the hundred patients reported that on the low-calorie diet they developed symptoms of "nervousness" or "weakness." Other complaints included irritability (eight people) and nausea (four people). Emotional disturbances were not studied, but four patients who reduced reported mounting tension during the diet period. One of the four developed a schizophrenic reaction.

What these and other similar studies indicated when I first saw them was that the medical profession was backward in its treatment of obesity. There is other evidence, too, in the profusion of people who are not physicians yet who can make a living treating, or claiming to treat, obesity. Not all of these people are quacks, but some are. And quacks can thrive only when orthodox medicine fails. You don't go to a quack to have a broken leg set. You go to an orthopedist, because you know that the orthopedist will be successful. You don't ask a quack to remove your appendix. You ask a surgeon, because you know that he can do the job quickly and well. People go to quacks only out of desperation. There are many quacks

83

in the field of nutrition because there are many desper-
ately obese people who have been to numerous doctors
and have remained obese.

The medical profession is too embroiled in conflicting
theories of obesity to recommend a single, successful
diet. There has been no standard diet, successful or
otherwise. While research into obesity proceeds, the treatment of obesity remains, for the most part, in the hands
of nonmedical specialists. There are more obese people in
the world today than ever before and, to paraphrase a
well-known statement, never before has so little been
known about so much.

Of course people flocked to low-calorie diets. Their
physicians, ignorant of the true cause of obesity, usually
approved and seldom disapproved. "Try it and be careful," many physicians said. There was nothing more
they could say. Some, perhaps, felt that a gland malfunc-
tion, yet unknown, was the true cause of obesity. Others
may have had other theories. But no one was sure, and
often the low-calorie diet was prescribed routinely—
there was nothing else to prescribe. At least one physician,
Dr. George L. Thorpe, faults the medical profession as a
whole for its treatment of obesity. "Doctors," Dr. Thorpe
suggests, "have been so preoccupied with the problems
of trauma and disease that they have ignored the public's
growing interest in the problem of excess weight." Wherever the fault may lie, the result probably is that you,
before reading this book, believed that "somehow or

other" low-calorie diets helped people to lose weight.

The sad fallacy is that, somehow or other, they don't— although the fallacy has been spread by every conceivable means. It has been reinforced by advertising, by the news media, by books, by word of mouth, by every means except the one that matters. That would be a proven record of effectiveness.

I have taken this effort to show the popularity and the failure of low-calorie programs because they represent a dietary pattern that is firmly established. I don't imagine that it will be easy to break, although I can often break it for my patients with one question: "Has a low-calorie diet worked for you?" "No," they say. They would not be in my office if it had worked. Then they often want to know what went wrong. They insist that they did not cheat, that they followed a diet given to them, often by a responsible medical man. Still the fat remains. What's wrong?

I've already mentioned that all calories are not the same; the calories of carbohydrate and the calories of unsaturated vegetable oil work quite differently in the system. To understand the whole story, you must understand a little more about your own system.

The human body is a great protector of the status quo. It does not seem to want to change. On a bitter wintry day your body temperature will be virtually the same as it is in the middle of an August heat wave. As a body clings to its temperature, so it clings to its weight level.

We all know lean people who weigh the same week

after week, month after month, year after year. These people don't eat the same things each week. They don't take the same amount of exercise. But their body has found its natural weight; it is in a state called "caloric equilibrium." (This term has nothing to do with low-calorie diets. It means, in effect, that the body takes in and expends equal amounts of energy.)

Fat people reach an equilibrium, too. Despite what you may suppose or may have heard, the obese are not constantly gaining weight. They gain weight for months and years, but then they reach a plateau, albeit a plateau too high for comfort. They remain at the plateau for a time, perhaps for many years. Then, after a long period at, say, 250 pounds, they again resume gaining weight. This time they may put on an extra 30 pounds. Then they are at another plateau: 280. The pattern continues this way, but most fat people spend most of their time on these plateaus. Their periods of weight gain may be brief, if intense.

Over the years a lean man's appetite is balanced quite precisely to his needs. He eats as much as his body requires; he hungers for no more. The fat man on a plateau is in an identical situation; his appetite, too, is balanced to his bodily wants. Unfortunately, in the fat man's case his body wants to maintain its fat, for fat is part of its general status quo. The fat body does not always want to gain weight, but it never wants to lose.

Body balance is a remarkably precise thing. To maintain constant weight over a period of twenty years, which is what many lean people do, energy intake and energy expenditure must be almost identical. The margin for error is only one half of one per cent.

When your body is maintaining the status quo, it may be said to be static. When it is gaining weight *or when it is losing weight*, the body is dynamic. When you put yourself on a low-calorie diet, you are disturbing the balance of forces within your body. By sharply limiting your calorie intake, you are jarring the body out of its static state. You are making it dynamic again. You are taking in less energy than you expend.

But a body transformed from static to dynamic does not abruptly go back from dynamic to static. It remains dynamic for a time. So here, in practice, is what happens:

A fat man who has weighed 250 pounds for a year decides to shed weight by cutting calories. He succeeds in losing 20 pounds, a mere skirmish in his battle of the bulge—and large battles loom ahead. When he stops the diet, as he must because it is subnutritional, his body does not become static at 230 pounds. The diet has shoved him from his plateau; it has made his body dynamic. Now, on its normal bill of fare, his body responds in a manner that horrifies him. He gains and gains and gains. Before his body has become static again, he finds he weighs 265 pounds. Net result of the low-calorie diet: aggravation, fatigue and a weight gain of 15 pounds.

Here's another point and another case: The calorie faddists insist that by careful control of calorie intake weight can be controlled; that is, by balancing the energy you get from food with the energy you expend, your weight will remain the same. What's wrong with this supposition is that no such balance is really possible unless the body itself establishes it—and when the body establishes it, there is no problem of weight gain.

Consider a man 5 feet 10 inches tall, who at the age of thirty weighs 160 pounds, a weight that statistics tell us is normal. Twenty years later, at the age of fifty, he has gained 40 pounds and weighs 200. (Statistics here tell us that this weight gain has increased his chances of early death by 45 per cent.)

Now examine this man's weight gain closely. Forty pounds over twenty years is an average weight gain of 2 pounds a year. We know, of course, that he did not gain evenly, that he went from plateau to plateau, but the average is important to this point. Expressed as calories, an average gain of 2 pounds a year means that 8,172 calories are stored as fat. That's 23 calories a day—in other words, *one small glass of tomato juice.*

Can it be argued that if this man had taken in 23 fewer calories a day for twenty years he would not have gained weight? Can it be supposed that a diet could have been worked out so precisely that it matched his requirements to the calorie? The answer to both questions is no. Besides, neither question cuts to the core of the problem. For the crux of the matter is not how many calories he took in, but what his body did with those calories.

Sometimes, when he was at a plateau, his body handled its calorie intake properly. Other times, when he was moving up from one plateau to a higher one, his body lost that ability. We cannot anticipate these bodily changes. We can't fool the body. The key question, then, is, What produced these occasional imbalances in the man's system? Low-calorie diets offer no answers. Worse, they are not even effective treatment.

Let me, then, finally describe, in the light of current medical knowledge and my own research, what's wrong with that popular, persistent humbug called the low-calorie diet:

1. It is not effective. You may not lose any weight at all. If you do lose, you may lose more vital body tissue than you lose fat.

2. It is not harmless. Your body wants to maintain itself. When you or a nutrition expert try to outsmart your body by providing it with less energy than it expends, your body will react. It may react mildly; you feel weak and irritable. It may react violently. There are cases of deaths caused by repeated reliance on crash programs built around low-calorie diets.

3. It is temporary. No one can long sustain himself on insufficient food. Sooner or later his body's demand—hunger—will force him off his low-calorie program. The low-calorie diet is temporary; the problem of obesity is permanent.

4. It is based on incorrect ideas. All calories, you remember, are not the same. Most low-calorie diets seem to say a calorie is a calorie is a calorie. But the body is not fooled. It persists in differentiating between calories

89

of carbohydrate, fat and protein. Because the basic idea is incorrect, a low-calorie, high-carbohydrate diet is likely not only to fail, but to make you add poundage.

5. It upsets a delicate body mechanism. By throwing a static body into a dynamic state we are starting a chain reaction and we do not know where it will end—except that it usually ends in extra weight.

6. It does not affect the cause of obesity. As a result, it can never be a cure, at best only a treatment.

7. It doesn't work. There are some rare cases in which a low-calorie diet has produced the desired weight loss, fewer still in which it produced a weight loss the patient could sustain. For the overwhelming majority of us, low-calorie diets fail.

I can understand, in view of the tremendous popularity low-calorie diets have enjoyed over the past few decades, why it may be difficult for you suddenly to accept the fact that these diets are nothing more than medical and nutritional failures. Think it over. Consider the evidence. Remember that medicine moves forward, that old and baffling medical riddles are being solved all the time. Then discard low-calorie diets as a treatment for obesity the way our ancestors discarded amulets as a treatment for fever. For the amulet and the low-calorie diet now properly belong to times that are past.

# CHAPTER SIX

# WHY YOU

# GET FAT

SOME OF THE EARLIEST EVIDENCE that I had discovered the prime cause of obesity appeared, or disappeared, in the delivery room of the New York City hospital where I am an attending physician.

When a baby is born in a modern hospital, of course, the obstetrician does not work alone. Anesthetists, residents, interns, nurses and sometimes other attending physicians assist. As my weight began to drop and my waist began to shrink, the people with whom I worked in the delivery room were curious. Some of them had weight problems themselves.

After I explained my new nutrition principle, fat began to vanish from the delivery-room staff. In all, I estimate that, counting all hands, some 800 pounds were lost over a period of months. Word of this spread through the hospital and one day a portly, distinguished physician whom I knew said that he wanted to talk to me.

"I didn't believe," he said, "but, all right, I'm convinced. The evidence in the hospital has convinced me."

"What do you want me to do?" I asked.

"Tell me how to lose weight," this physician said.

"The principle," I began, "is based—"

"Never mind the principle," he said. "Just tell me what I should eat."

Perhaps you feel the same way. Perhaps you think, "I don't care why I'm fat. I just want to know how to be lean." If an obese physician feels this way, I can understand why many of my patients do, too. But other patients, and most physicians, want to know as much as they can about the bodily processes which produce fat. It is a reasonable curiosity, but not one that can be satisfied simply. The production of fat is a complex process; explaining it involves a certain complexity. You can, of course, simply skip the explanation and proceed to the new nutrition principle itself, which we shall do after this chapter and the next. But I think it is a good idea to make a serious effort to understand the process of fat production. Then you will not only understand what you must do to lose weight, you will understand why you are doing it.

I worked for a long time in laboratories studying, analyzing and reasoning before I reached my conclusions. They are the results of considerable effort, but the response has more than made up for my pains. I have experienced the joy of seeing my patients with "hopeless" obesity problems lose weight, week after week, and gain first hope and then more happiness than they had experienced for years. I have received enthusiastic responses from physicians in the United States, in Canada and in England, after my papers on obesity appeared in professional journals. As I say, hard work, but a happy ending.

Let's look at this question, unanswered for centuries: What is it that makes people fat? The underlying reason, in more than 95 per cent of all cases of obesity, is an imbalance between energy output and energy intake. That is, the body, in carrying out its functions, does not expend as many work units as it takes in through foods and liquids. This is a disturbance in the metabolism, and it shows up in three ways:

1. The body forms fat at a rate that is faster than normal.

2. The body *stores* fat at a rate that is faster than normal. Fat formed in the digestive system quickly reaches the arms, the thighs, in the form of fat deposits— the deposits that stretch your skin and distort your shape.

3. The body disposes of stored fat at a rate that is slower than normal. This is why it is so difficult to lose weight from the places you want to lose it. The body that is forming and storing fat fast can't get rid of the fat already stored as easily as it should—*regardless of how carefully you count calories*. The metabolic disturbance works on you in three ways, all damaging.

When you understand that obesity is caused by metabolic disturbance, you also understand something else.

93

All the talk about glandular conditions has been over-emphasized. "She's fat because of her glands," you have undoubtedly heard people say. Actually, only five persons in every hundred—one in twenty—who suffer from obesity are fat because of their glands. Instead of concerning ourselves with this small minority, we'll do better to examine the dominant issue, the whole question of metabolism and fat.

Metabolism is simply a term for the chemical workings of a body. When you are resting, your metabolism is at its minimum, which you may know as the basal metabolic rate, or by the initials BMR. The basal metabolic rate is measured by a test performed on the patient when his stomach is empty—when his digestive system is not working on food. The easiest way to administer the test is to have the patient lie on a comfortable bed, in a room that is warm and quiet, and keep him there for at least half an hour, so that the muscles become completely relaxed; a mask is then put over his face and he breathes pure oxygen. (As you know, we take oxygen from the air and in the metabolic process convert it into carbon dioxide.) Then the amount of carbon dioxide the patient produces is measured, and from this the basal metabolic rate is calculated. This is a sure, certain test. The more rapidly your body functions, the more carbon dioxide it produces. The slower it functions, the less carbon dioxide it produces. Carbon dioxide is a perfect index to the body's chemical workings. What are these workings exactly? Some of the food we eat and the liquid is converted into energy. The rest, aside from waste, is distributed through the blood stream to all the tissues of the body, for growth and for repair. This is the metabolic process—something vital to existence, something that cannot function without oxygen.

Your basal metabolic rate represents the minimum number of work units your body needs to sustain all its vital functions during rest. For the average man, the minimum is 1,700 units; for the average woman, the figure is 1,300. Bear in mind that these are absolute minimums.

What does the average person need to sustain ordinary activities? The Food and Agriculture Organization of the United Nations recently recommended work-unit requirements for what they called a "reference" man and a "reference" woman. The U.N.'s reference man is twenty-five years old and healthy. He lives in a temperate climate and he neither gains nor loses weight. His activities include eight hours a day of moderate work, four hours of sedentary activity. He is out of doors for two hours and walks about five miles during the course of a day. He weighs about 145 pounds. This man, the U.N. organization reports, needs to take in 3,200 work units a day to sustain himself.

The reference woman also is twenty-five years old and a healthy resident of the temperate zone. She does either housework or light industrial work and she weighs about 120 pounds. Her requirement is 2,300 work units to continue functioning properly.

You will often see these work units referred to as

calories, which is a perfectly proper term. I prefer to call them work units because of all the confusion about calories over the last decades. For the normal person, calories of fat, protein or carbohydrate seem to have about the same effect on weight. The normal person, the one whose body maintains caloric equilibrium, has not had to concern himself with what type of calories he took in. (Although medical discoveries of the past few years indicate that even a thin person may shorten his life by eating too high a proportion of carbohydrates.) But for the obese person, let me repeat, all calories are not the same. So *work unit* seems to me a safer term.

You are probably quite familiar with basal metabolism. Perhaps a relative or friend has undergone a basal-metabolism test, or perhaps you yourself have. But just as important to an understanding of why obese people are heavy is what we call "total metabolism." Basal metabolism measures a comfortable, relaxed, resting, fasting individual. Except in the final hours of a good night's sleep, few of us can be described as comfortable, relaxed, resting and fasting. Whenever we eat, play, work, walk, whenever we feel tension, the rate of our metabolism changes. This increased metabolic rate goes into creating our total metabolism. So our total metabolism is our basal metabolism *plus* the extra heat produced—the energy required to move, digest, hit a tennis ball, squirm in an uncomfortable chair, work up the courage to ask for a raise or simply to worry.

As you recall from the discussion of skipping meals, food alone increases the metabolism. About an hour after a meal, the metabolic rate begins to rise. Three hours later it is at a peak. Then it decreases toward a fasting level, hitting bottom between the sixth and the eighth hour after a meal. Carbohydrate and fat cause the least rise in the rate. Protein causes the greatest. Instinctively we eat less meat during a spell of hot weather. Instinctively, too, people living in tropical climates do not eat very much meat. They concentrate on fats and carbohydrates. Arabs, for example, sometimes chew chunks of pure fat when scorching heat strikes the desert. Many races in the tropics eat large quantities of cereals and fats. It is a rare tropical man who likes lean meat—rare and also hot.

Exercise—all types of muscular activity—is what increases our expenditure of work units most sharply. But extremes of climate can have a strong effect, too. Why? The answer goes back to the body's continual attempt to maintain its status quo. In this case, it is a question of maintaining body temperature.

When you run hard, or labor hard, you are taking work units from the body that would ordinarily be converted into heat. The body wants to maintain itself at 98.6 degrees, and to do this when you are active it must produce many more work units than it does when you are resting. Similarly, on a cold day it must produce more work units to maintain the 98.6 than it needs on a hot day in summer.

Within the body is something rather like a thermostat.

Set a thermostat at 70 and in January, when the temperature dips below the freezing point, your home heating system will work long and hard to maintain a comfortable temperature in your house. On a day in April, when it is much warmer, the home heating system will work only infrequently. On a day in summer it probably will not have to work at all. If you've paid the bills for a home heating system, you know that the consumption of fuel— oil, coal or gas—varies sharply with the amount of work the system must do to maintain 70 degrees. (And you hope for nice warm winters.) The body too consumes fuel in its metabolic process at sharply varying rates.

The fuel for a home heating system consists of fairly simple molecules and the heat is produced by the process of burning. What is the body's fuel? The food you eat, the liquids you drink, the air you breathe and, sometimes, the tissues stored in your body. To lose fat, you must make your body consume its stored fat, a process my new nutrition principle achieves.

Your body is more complex than your heating system. It takes the complicated molecules of food and through the complicated process of digestion converts them into energy. What it does ultimately is extract the carbon and the hydrogen from your food and combine them with the oxygen you breathe. This process, called oxidation, results in an even, steady flow of energy. (Coal burning is oxidation, too, but the body controls oxidation far more precisely than does a furnace.) In a healthy, lean person, the energy is sufficient to provide the strength he needs for his activities as well as to provide the heat he needs for a 98.6 body temperature. Sufficient, but no more. His system is not clogged with surpluses. This is the working of a balanced body, a normal metabolism.

For more than half a century physicians and medical research workers have studied metabolism and obesity. Sometimes they came close to the truth. One physician years ago stated of people who were in a prediabetic state, "Obese individuals of this type have already an altered metabolism for sugar, but instead of excreting the sugar in the urine they transfer it to fat-producing parts of the body whose tissues are well prepared to receive it." This was close, but then the physician abandoned his research. Until comparatively recently there was no laboratory technique known to check out the theories of metabolism of obese people. So the cause of fat remained a mystery and all treatments began in the dark. Based on uncheckable theories, the treatment failed.

Even something as widely employed as the basal-metabolism test provided an incorrect picture. According to the standard test of BMR, most obese persons have normal metabolism. This test uses as a measuring rod a person's total area of skin surface. Why? Because when metabolic knowledge was incomplete, one thing physicians did know was this: Throughout all the animal kingdom there is a constant mathematical relationship between an animal's energy output and the surface area of its body. We knew that animals, on their own, were not afflicted with obesity. (Have you ever seen a fat giraffe?) Very well. Their metabolic rate varied with skin surface, and they weren't obese. What works for a giraffe might work for a human.

Later we learned more about animals, and about humans. We found that just as there is a constant relationship between an animal's energy output and his surface area, there also exists a relationship between energy output and weight. And this was tremendously important. For where a large person or a large giraffe will produce more energy than a small one in *exact proportion* to the increased area of skin, a fat person will not produce more energy than a lean one in proportion to his weight.

Of course, a fat 200-pounder produces more energy than a lean man of 165 pounds. He has to in order to keep functioning—his body has to if it is to maintain status quo. But he will not produce as much more energy as he should. Although the lean man produces the same amount of energy for each square inch of skin, he gets more pep per pound than does the fat man.

Undoubtedly any basal-metabolism test you have taken was based on your skin area, not your weight. What private hopes you may have had that a metabolism test would help get at the cause of your obesity probably vanished when you learned your metabolism was about normal.

A medical argument still persists about whether skin area or total weight is the proper criterion for calculating basal metabolism. For metabolic disturbances not connected with obesity, the skin area system is superior. But for getting at the cause of obesity, the skin area formula is valueless. There will be no sign of a fat person's metabolic disturbance in a standard basal-metabolism test.

What, then, is the metabolic disturbance that makes fat people heavy? The disturbance involves a substance of which you probably know little. It is pyruvic acid, one of the many complex substances the body produces as it converts food to energy.

In a person with normal metabolism, food, liquid and air are converted into energy and such tissues as the body needs to maintain its normal state. Carbohydrates—the sugars and starches in our diet—ultimately are broken down to energy, carbon dioxide and water. This is not a simple matter, like burning oil or coal. As the carbohydrates are broken down they go through numerous changes, and in one change they become pyruvic acid.

The pyruvic acid accumulates within an obese person's system and the results are unfortunate on two counts:

1. Pyruvic acid acts as an inhibitor on the body's ability to get rid of stored fat. With an excess of pyruvic acid in your system, the fat you store stays stored. You can't get rid of it.

2. Pyruvic acid itself ultimately is converted into fat. Here complicated enzyme processes are involved. After these processes have worked and converted pyruvic acid into substances called neutral fats, or glycerides, the neutral fats are deposited into your adipose, or fat, tissue.

101

In other words, pyruvic acid ends up as a deposit of fat in a place where you are probably already fat enough, or long since too fat.

Clearly, then, anyone who is fat wants to limit sharply the amount of pyruvic acid in his system. How? Pryuvic acid is produced from carbohydrates, so anyone with an obesity problem should limit sharply the amount of carbohydrates he consumes. But there is no need to limit the amount of protein the person eats, nor is there any need to limit the fat, provided the fat is the right kind.

The right kind of fat is vitally important. With it, a high-fat diet is far more effective than a high-protein diet in losing weight. The body which is lightly supplied with carbohydrates will burn some of its stored fat as fuel. By eating large quantities of fat you set in motion a process which stimulates the pituitary gland and gets this fat burning going at a higher rate.

Here at last is something fortunate for the obese. A thin person eating a high-fat diet will burn fat at a slightly greater rate than he would otherwise. His body is preserving its status quo. As he eats more fat, his body burns fat more rapidly to dispose of the extra fat he eats. But an obese person eating large quantities of fat is stimulated to burn fat three times as strongly as a lean person. The obese person not only burns the fat he eats; his system gets so fired up that it burns the fat he has accumulated over the years. And that, of course, is the idea—the basis of sensible weight reduction.

On a proper high-fat diet you not only don't gain

weight, you *lose* weight. You lose and you continue to lose until your body reaches its normal weight. Then you stop losing, because your body will adjust; it will burn fat not at a fat man's rate but at a normal rate. More than 95 per cent of all obese people who bring their bodies down to normal on a high-fat diet find their bodies remain normal. But understand, this is a treatment and not a cure. You must continue to follow the high-fat program. Return to carbohydrates and once again you will accumulate poundage. But following the program is not difficult. On a high-fat diet you can eat as much as you want—as many steaks and chops as any hungry man could ask.

Because my new nutrition principle involves a certain change in your eating habits that you must follow for all your days, I call it a way of life. I think you will find it a pleasant way when you have tried it.

I stress metabolism first because it is most important. Once you comprehend the villainous role of pyruvic acid and the heroic role of the right kind of fats, you understand why a diet that is rich in carbohydrates may make you gain, whatever its calorie content, and why a diet rich in the right kind of fats will make you lose. But, as there is more to your body functioning than metabolic rate, there is more to understanding the causes of obesity than the existence of pyruvic acid.

A term to know is *lipo-equilibrium. Lipid* is a general medical word for a fat, and *equilibrium,* of course, refers to balance. A body in lipo-equilibrium maintains a nor-

103

mal level of fat, no more and no less. This requires a sort of co-operation between your liver and the fat deposits about your body.

Fat is formed in only two ways. Either the liver produces it or fatty tissue produces it. Fat tissue tends to create more fat tissue. The more fat you have, the more fat you can create. (I imagine some fat people suspect this already; they may be interested to discover this medical confirmation of their belief.)

But fat is broken down only one way—by the liver. The liver takes a complex fat and breaks it down to a simpler substance which the body can use for energy. The liver here acts like a railroad fireman who breaks coal into chunks, which the furnace can then use to drive the engine. Without the liver your body could make no use of fat, which is one reason why the liver is essential to life.

Your lipo-equilibrium, this balance between fat formation and fat disposal, is controlled, as we have seen, by your carbohydrate metabolism. This is the point to which nearly all fat people can trace their trouble. But there are other influences upon this balance, too. This includes the metabolism of your adipose tissue—how rapidly your fat creates more fat. It also includes the functioning of your central nervous system and the secretions of certain glands.

When any or all of these forces go out of order, your lipo-equilibrium is disturbed. Something, usually a person's inability to handle carbohydrates, breaks down and he begins producing an excess of fat. Why doesn't the liver go to work on this extra fat? It tries to, but the liver is a limited organ. Its ability to break down fat is limited. So despite the best efforts of your liver, fat builds up in the body faster than it can be disposed of. It collects in the body, most heavily in those areas already fat. As long as this disturbance continues, as long as the body creates fat faster than the liver can get rid of it, you will get fatter and fatter.

The problem here is difficult. Since fat makes fat, the fatter you are the more extra fat you can produce. And the more extra fat you produce, the greater the body's capacity to produce still more fat. Further, not all fat is the same. Analyzing fat tissue taken from obese people and from lean people clearly demonstrates that the fat on fat men is harder, tougher, than the fat which a lean man carries. What this means is that fat on a fat man is more concentrated; it contains less water. (I have made actual measurements of this.)

The fat man's fat is extremely difficult for his body to break down. It is his hard fat, fat which has been evident as a paunch or as a bulging neck for some years, which lingers longest, even on a successful reducing program. New fat, even on a fat man, is comparatively soft to the touch. It is fairly easy for the body to mobilize this fat and, through the action of the liver, break it down. But fat that a fat man or woman has carried for a long time is hard to the touch and equivalently hard for the body to utilize.

Have you ever noticed how people on a low-calorie diet

105

sometimes grow gaunt-faced while, say, their upper arms, which have been fat for a long time, seem to remain just as heavy as ever? This is not an illusion. The body, not getting enough fuel from a low-calorie diet, turns to what reserves it can muster. Obtaining energy from vital muscle tissue about the face and neck may be far easier for the body than obtaining energy from the tough, hard, long-entrenched fat on the upper arms. The body gets its energy as best it can. The dieter loses weight, but does not lose much fat, and he loses almost no fat from the places where it is most unsightly and, possibly, the greatest threat to his health.

Just how obese you become depends on how extensive is the disturbance to your lipo-equilibrium. On later pages we can discuss the development of a diet engineered precisely to a weakness in the carbohydrate metabolism, the overwhelming cause of obesity. But other causes of obesity are possible, if rare, and you should be aware of them. If one of these other causes seems to fit you, discuss the matter with your physician. I think we had better take these other disturbances singly:

*Disturbances of the Central Nervous System.* We have evidence that certain conditions of the outer layer of the brain, the cerebral cortex, cause a sluggishness in body functions. This sluggishness then causes a decrease in your energy output. Fat that should be burned is not. It is stockpiled by the body. Problems involving the cerebral cortex are not common and can be determined only by a physician.

106

Other conditions, which you can recognize easily, cause disturbances, too. Excess excitement or stress may over-stimulate the trunk-line nerve center which, oddly enough, makes you crave certain foods, particularly sweets, which are rich in carbohydrates. What sort of conditions can do this? Almost any that are extreme enough. A crisis at home or in business; the loss of a job or an unwanted transfer to a strange city; a broken love affair or the stormy beginning of another. Such stress, by affecting the trunk-line nerve center, upsets the lipo-equilibrium. If you see a person suddenly begin wolfing down candy and second helpings of pie and chocolate cake, he may not nec-essarily be a hog; he may be emotionally disturbed or on the brink of a crisis.

It would be pleasant if such people solved their crises and returned to normal weight. But they do not always solve them; some seem to live in a state of continual crisis, and further, even if they do solve them, the solu-tion may come too late to help cure their new obesity. Re-member that fat creates more fat and that the body works to sustain the status quo. Many people who grow obese at a time of stress are triggering a chain reaction which they cannot reverse. My nutrition principle can bring them back to their proper weight, but, of course, if they move from one emotional crisis to another, and their trunk-line nerve center responds by producing a craving for sweets, their problem involves other aspects. Again I find myself like the man in Chile who could make an excellent rain-coat but could do nothing about the rain.

I want to stress that a nervous craving for sweets that has organic origin is not common. Because you have read about it, do not feel free to say to yourself, "Well, it's been a tough day and I'm all upset. Guess I'll have a few helpings of ice cream." The one is a clinical condition; the other is a case of a different sort—a case of someone looking for an excuse. Before you look for an excuse, I suggest you re-examine Chapter Three to see what obesity does to your health and to your life expectancy. You will almost certainly conclude that while it has been a rough day, you don't really need those helpings of ice cream. Some cheese, low in carbohydrate, will do instead.

*Disturbances of the Endocrine Glands.* The endocrines, or ductless hormone-secreting glands, are a hard-working bunch—the pituitary, the thyroid, the pancreas and the adrenals. They work together, as a unit, or individually, in order to control the metabolism of your body. Their functions are so closely associated that damage to one of these glands can disturb the balance of your entire hormone system.

The endocrine glands have neither ducts nor tubes. The hormones they produce are fed directly into the blood stream, which, of course, reaches the entire body.

Since the endocrines affect both mind and body, they affect everything. In a proper nutritional pattern, their hormones help maintain the lipo-equilibrium. Let's see how each of the endocrines relates to the problem of obesity.

The *pituitary* is a tiny gland situated at the base of the brain. It is fashioned of three lobes, but in all it weighs

108

only a little more than an aspirin tablet. The pituitary is, among other things, the supervisor of hormone production in your body. It produces hormones which work on other glands, such as the thyroid and the sex glands. It also produces two hormones which directly affect the manner in which the system utilizes fat.

One of these pituitary hormones promotes the deposit of fat in fat cells. The other stimulates the release of fat from fat cells. When you produce these hormones in proper amounts, your body's equilibrium is more likely to be maintained. When you produce these hormones in quantities that do not match, there will be trouble, probably in the shape of obesity.

Most obese people have no pituitary disturbance, but it is important to know that for some, however few, a pituitary disturbance *may* be the cause of obesity.

The *thyroid* gland is located in the neck, directly in front of the windpipe. Under the control of the pituitary, it secretes a hormone called thyroxin, which is rich in iodine and which helps the body burn up fat. If your thyroid is particularly active you reduce fat to water and carbon dioxide much more quickly. If the thyroid is inactive, the fat turnover is slowed. Then you are likely to be nervous, drowsy, irritable, tired; you are not getting the fuel you need to keep going. Since less fat is burned, more fat is stored. An underactive thyroid can produce obesity.

The *pancreas*, which is located in the back of the stomach, is usually one of the first of the delicate body mechanisms that deteriorate under the strain of a diet too rich in sugar and starches. The main function of the pancreas is the secretion of insulin, a substance which is vital in the control of fat formation. Among other things, insulin speeds up the body's transformation of carbohydrates into fat. It also works on the storing of this fat and inhibits the release of fat already stored. As you can see, the role which insulin fills tends to make you put on fat. How much insulin will your pancreas produce? In a normal person the amount varies with his intake of carbohydrates; the more carbohydrates he eats, the more insulin his pancreas produces. By controlling carbohydrate intake, the normal person controls his own production of insulin. This is another point against eating a large proportion of carbohydrates in your diet.

The *adrenals* are two peanut-sized glands, lying just above the kidneys, which produce at least twenty important body substances, including cortisone. You cannot live without your adrenal glands. Removal of five sixths of the shell, or cortex, of the adrenals results in death within a few days.

Overactive adrenal glands cause a disease called Cushing's syndrome, which creates a unique pattern of fat. A victim of Cushing's syndrome puts on excessive fat over the spine, the upper chest, the hips and, most notably, the cheeks. The first things you notice about someone suffering from Cushing's syndrome are the jowls. They sag under the burden of a large quantity of extra fat. Even

110

R.D.

1,200 calories a day if you're a woman, 1,800 calories if you're a man, and you're in good health. You also may wish to join mutual support groups, such as TOPS, Weight Watchers, or Diet Workshop, since it seems easier to battle the bulge when you have company in your misery. Many hospitals and hospital-connected health centers also have developed weight control programs as a public health service.

Whatever diet you adopt, there are three essentials to keep in mind: The first consideration, of course, is the number of calories. If the amount you eat is not restricted in one way or another, there can be no weight loss. A reducing diet that goes below 1,200 calories for women and 1,800 for men may not be adequate in essential nutrients no matter how well-balanced the menus. There just is not enough food allowed. And diets (for women) which call for only 800 calories a day often produce adverse effects on body metabolism. They should not be used without careful medical supervision.

DIETS DEPEND ON a wide variety of techniques to be successful. Most aim to modify the number of calories prescribed by placing conditions on eating. For example, some purposefully unbalance the proportion of protein to fat to carbohydrate they recommend. The average American diet contains 12 to 14

...om protein, about 42 ... 46 per cent from ...alth reasons, we can ...nsumption of complex ...ed sugars) to about 58 ...l consumption of fat to about 30 per cent. But to unbalance your normal diet by increasing or decreasing one of these nutrients by one-half or more not only makes it more difficult for the dieter to eat usual foods but, if the diet is low in carbohydrates, the body's water balance will be upset. Thus, a great part of the weight lost in the initial stages will be body water, not fat.

Some diet plans may specify each and every food or, as with the "grapefruit" diet, focus on one or two foods. Some diets also specify particular conditions for eating, such as drinking large amounts of water — or tomato or grapefruit juice or unspecified amounts of alcohol!

The basis of many of the more successful diet programs today is behavior modification. Many others borrow the techniques of these programs, which are not only helpful while dieting but for maintaining the weight loss once it is off. Some popular examples are vigorous exercise, use of yoga to relax and reduce some of the stress associated with dieting, instructions to eat slowly or only in a certain place or under certain conditions. Food diaries which record all that is eaten are also helpful. But whatever the support technique used, pick one that is compatible with your way of life.

Last but no less in importance is the matter of nutritional adequacy. Does the daily fare include a prudent serving of food from each of

the following basic seven food groups?

Group 1: One or more servings of a leafy, green or yellow vegetable.

Group 2: One or more servings of citrus fruits, tomatoes, raw cabbage, or salad.

Group 3: Two servings chosen from all the fruits and vegetables not included in groups one and two.

Group 4: Two or more servings of fortified milk or its equivalent in cheese or yogurt.

Group 5: One or two servings of lean meat or poultry, fish, dried beans, peas or nuts, and (especially for children and young women) eggs.

Group 6: At least two and preferably four servings of grain or other cereal products and a slice of whole grain or enriched bread.

Group 7: Depending on calories, butter or fortified margarine or salad oils may be allowed in limited amounts. (Of all the nutrients, fat is the highest in calories, ounce for ounce, so use it sparingly.)

So there it is. If a diet that you have seen in a magazine, newspaper, or book meets all these criteria, then go ahead and try it. If you do not like it, you can always fall back on the sure-fire way: Eat less and exercise more.

Q — During the winter months, one of the most popular snacks in our house is freshly popped corn. My kids certainly enjoy it even without salt and butter, and it certainly is one of the least expensive snacks I can provide. But does popcorn provide any nutrients except calories?

A — If you're thinking of popcorn solely in terms of nutrients, forget it. It does provide a little protein, small amounts of B vitamins, and a bit of iron. But hardly enough to add popcorn to your diet.

Nonetheless, popcorn does have several things to recommend it. As you point out, it certainly is an inexpensive snack food. In addition, if eaten without butter or margarine it is really quite low in calories, making it a good choice for anyone who is a weight watcher. A whole cup of popped corn contains only 25 calories, less than half as many as in a single slice of bread and only about one-fourth the number in a small cake-type doughnut. Finally, dentists often suggest popcorn, as a snack food because it contains no sugar and therefore is far less likely to contribute to tooth decay.

Liquor items available only at licensed Chicago and suburban (Illinois) stores with liquor departments. Prices subject to state and local taxes, if cable.

**Osco liquor**

**Gordon's Gin**
1.75 liters
(59.2 ounces).

Osco Sale Price

**8²⁹**

**Sasha Vodka**
1.75 liters
(59.2 ounces).

Osco Sale Price

**6⁴⁹**

**Calvert Extra Blend**
1.75 liters
(59.2 ounces).

Osco Sale Price

**8⁹⁹**

**Early Times Bourbon**
1.75 liters
(59.2 ounces)

Osco Sale Price

**9⁶⁹**

when a victim of Cushing's syndrome becomes generally emaciated, he retains much of his fat in the characteristic places. This is a case of pure glandular obesity, a condition which cannot be controlled by diet. But, fortunately, this disease is rare.

The *sex glands* too play some role in obesity, particularly in governing the distribution of fat. We know that where a man will acquire fat at the back of his neck and at his waist, a woman will acquire it in the buttocks and on the thighs. (These are common, but not unvarying, patterns.) If a man suffers from a disease or undergoes an accident necessitating the removal of his testicles, his fat distribution will become feminine; that is, he will put on fat in the buttocks and on the thighs. He will also be likely to put on more over-all fat. A woman whose ovaries have been removed similarly tends to become fat.

The sex glands have a role in a small minority of obesity cases.

I want to repeat that the role of glands in obesity has been overemphasized for years. More than 95 per cent of the Americans who are obese have healthy, well-functioning glands, so if you are obese it is almost certainly in spite of, not because of, your glands.

The cause of your problem almost certainly lies in your metabolism—not in a fault detectable in the standard basal-metabolism test, but in a fault that was discovered only after years of research in laboratories.

111

The fat burned by your body burns clean and hot. The carbohydrates are what your metabolism burns improperly. Instead of converting them to energy, carbon dioxide and water, it converts some of them only to the substance called pyruvic acid. And later pyruvic acid becomes fat. How to eliminate pyruvic acid? Cut down on carbohydrates. A major point in my new nutrition principle is a sharp limiting of the carbohydrate foods you eat. On pages 137–47, in Chapter Eight, you will find a table listing the carbohydrate content of all the foods Americans eat.

# CHAPTER SEVEN

# THE ROLE OF FOOD

WHAT IS FOOD for you? The question seems absurdly simple. Food is for energy, for growth and for the maintenance of the human body. Yet the manner in which your body handles food is one of the most complicated processes in the world. Even now we do not know everything about the process. We cannot reproduce it in all its complexity, nor can we explain it as precisely as we can explain the workings of an automobile engine.

Still, we have made great strides. We now understand enough of the role each food plays to determine how much and what food you should eat. I think in surveying our foods we ought to begin with the carbohydrates. The best way to begin your battle of the bulge is to know your enemy.

Carbohydrates are an important part of a good nutritional pattern, but they should be consumed only in moderation. Eaten moderately, they add important roughage to your diet. And, of course, many carbohydrates are tasty. There is no point in ignoring the importance of taste. We all like to eat foods that taste good.

113

But too high a concentration of carbohydrates is the cause of millions upon millions of cases of obesity. It is an unavoidable, if unpleasant, fact that the average American eats more carbohydrates than he should.

What, exactly, are carbohydrates? The table on pages 137–47 lists them all. One example is sugar—and the average American now consumes 150 pounds of white refined sugar each year. That's triple the average consumption in the days before World War I. Products of bleached (white) flour—bread, cakes—are also prime sources of carbohydrates. So are polished rice—the white rice most Americans eat—and corn and oats and dates and raisins and prunes and figs and liquor, and many vegetables and fruits. Most food, of course, contains a great deal of water. Discounting the water, the foods that I have listed are almost entirely carbohydrate.

These are the carbohydrates you eat. Within the body, after the body chemistry has come into play, carbohydrates are found in two forms. One is called glucose, and this is found in the blood stream. Perhaps after surgery you have been given glucose intravenously, from a bottle supported over your bed. This is because glucose is important in warding off shock, or in countering its effects. The other bodily form of carbohydrates is a substance called glycogen, which is primarily found in the liver. Your body can easily convert glycogen into glucose. Counting them both, the glucose and the glycogen, carbohydrates make up about one half of one per cent of normal body weight. No more. And remember that fat represents 11 per cent of normal body weight.

114

The total weight of carbohydrates in a normal body is 300 grams. A glass and a half of beer provides 300 grams of carbohydrate—all that the normal person needs. Further, your body can convert as much as 40 per cent of the protein you eat into carbohydrate. You do not have to fear that, in cutting down on carbohydrates, you will be endangering your body or putting any strain on it.

What happens when you eat and drink *more* carbohydrates than your body can use is the real problem. Some individuals are able to cope with excessive amounts of carbohydrates, at least as far as weight is concerned. But others are not. Among most obese people, the excess carbohydrates eventually are transformed into fat.

Your body tightly regulates the amount of glucose in the blood. Except under certain conditions and during certain illnesses, such as diabetes, the body regulates the blood sugar so that you are in no danger of suffering from the serious results of a disturbed sugar level. The intricate system of glands we mentioned in the previous chapter keeps the blood-sugar level constant, and so does something in your nervous system which no one has yet been able to define.

A French scientist once demonstrated that he could raise the level of blood sugar by injuring the brain; specifically, he punctured the floor of the fourth ventricle in the base of the brain. We do not, as I say, fully comprehend just why this is so, but we do know that both the brain and the glands work constantly to maintain normal blood-sugar level.

The body is a marvelous fabric of checks and counter-

115

checks, and a sudden drop in blood sugar is indeed serious. So the body guards against it very carefully. The accumulation of fat is less serious, at least initially. So here the body has no such careful safeguards, and obesity is a grave national problem while difficulties in maintaining blood-sugar level are, compared to obesity, rare.

It is important for you to understand that by cutting down on carbohydrates you are in no way endangering your health. You are, in fact, improving it. Carbohydrates contain no essential substances that the body must have to repair itself. The energy they provide, though quick, is limited. In excessive quantities they cause obesity. And, as we shall see in more detail later, the presence of too much carbohydrate in the system interferes with the proper use of fat.

Proteins are the second major element in food. They are vital. The word protein derives from the Greek *protos*, meaning "first," or "of first importance," and proteins are enormously important in keeping you healthy. They are the builders of the body; their role is often compared to that of bricks in a home. No bricks, no home. No proteins, no body.

Proteins affect your size and your weight. The primary sources of protein are meat and fish, and, since we eat a lot of meat, we are a nation of big men. Some interesting studies have been made of the relationship of protein to size.

In Australia, one study tells us, among people whose average protein intake is 18.1 grams a day the average height is almost 5 feet 8 inches, the average weight 169 pounds and the average life expectancy sixty-five years. In parts of Australia where the average protein intake is about ten grams, the average height is only a little over 5 feet 3 inches, the average weight is 127 pounds and the life expectancy also is lower than that of the other group.

In America, where our average consumption of protein is 25 grams a day, the average height is almost 5 feet 7 inches, the average weight 154 pounds and the average life expectancy sixty-four. For a dramatic contrast, we can turn to pre-Communist China. (No figures are available from Communist China, of course.) The average Chinese ate only 11 grams of protein a day. The average height was 5 feet 2 inches, the average weight 119 and the average life expectancy only thirty. Protein alone does not make anyone tall, husky and long-lived, nor does it entirely explain these striking statistical differences. But it is a major factor.

There has been some speculation about the effect of high temperatures on growth and physique. Some have theorized that man does not grow well in the tropics and pointed to several undersized tropical races as proof. But most tropical races are heavy eaters of vegetables and do not consume very much protein. The tropical races which are big meat eaters are large and strong. Examples are the Masai and Berber tribes of the Sahara, the Sudanese of Africa and the Punjabis of India. All these tribes number powerful, husky people among them, and all are bigger on the average than surrounding tribes which eat less meat and therefore consume smaller quantities of protein.

One old tradition about protein that stands up even today is its effect on sexual vigor. You have probably heard
mention of oysters and virility. The ancients believed that
oysters, fish and certain strong-flavored vegetables (actually, vegetables with a high protein content) were
aphrodisiac foods. The ancients believed these foods stimulated sexual activity. In a recent test a group of men
with normal sexual drives was fed a diet high in carbohydrates but low in proteins. Surprisingly quickly these
men began to lose interest in women. As part of the test,
the men were subjected to ordinarily stimulating experiences. Still they did not react. When they went back to
normal diets and began eating protein again, they picked
up where they had left off. Their sexual drive regained its
former intensity.

Protein is a combination of chemical substances called
amino acids. While protein, like a carbohydrate, contains
molecules of carbon, hydrogen and oxygen, protein also
contains nitrogen. The element nitrogen, which is essential to life, is not present in carbohydrates.

The body breaks down the protein you consume through
food into carbohydrates and into nitrogen. This protein
breakdown, as you remember, is one source of carbohydrates, and the typical American diet is so rich in protein
that many of us could probably subsist without eating any
carbohydrates at all. (I am not recommending that you
try. I am only pointing out that whereas you could not
live without protein, you could live, perhaps quite com-
fortably, without eating any sugars or starches.)

If the body turns protein into carbohydrate, you may wonder, won't it run into the problem of pyruvic acid? Won't obese people, in whom pyruvic acid turns to fat, get into as much weight trouble eating protein as they do eating carbohydrates? The answer, fortunately, is no. You can eat too much protein, just as you can eat too much carbohydrate. But practically you are not likely to. Your appetite is far better at regulating your protein intake than it is at regulating your carbohydrate intake. The problem of your eating so much protein that the body, in breaking down this protein, becomes oversupplied with carbohydrates is pretty much nonexistent.

Physiologists estimate that the body can use one gram of protein for every kilogram of body weight. Translating this into more meaningful terms, a 150-pounder can handle about 70 grams of protein a day. Two normal slices of good lean beef contain only 28 grams of protein. In practice, a 150-pounder is not likely to exceed his 70 grams very often or by very much.

The nitrogen in protein is particularly important:
1. To repair worn-out tissues. This process goes on constantly.
2. To form certain body defense mechanisms. These substances are significant in our ability to ward off a disease or to recover from a disease we have contracted.

For both these reasons, nitrogen is notably important to growing children, who are not only repairing worn tissue but also building longer, stronger bone and muscle. It is

119

vital to pregnant women and to anyone who is recovering from a prolonged or a serious illness.

When we consume more nitrogen, through the protein we eat, than we excrete through elimination, we are said to be in positive nitrogen balance. When we excrete more nitrogen than we consume, we are in negative nitrogen balance. You may not know these terms, but you can feel the difference.

When you starve yourself, or during some illnesses, you suffer the effects of negative nitrogen balance. Your body loses weight, but not necessarily fat. During negative nitrogen balance, your muscles, your kidneys, your liver and other organs become smaller. As a general rule, little fat is lost at first in starvation. If you starve or half starve yourself for a long time, you will eventually start losing considerable fat, but by that time you may have endangered your life. Someone who has maintained negative nitrogen balance through insufficient eating over a long period of time is less resistant to disease and is less likely to survive any serious disease he contracts. When you play with nitrogen you are playing with one of the wellsprings of life—a dangerous business, and one more argument against starving yourself or experimenting with a diet or formula that is subnutritional.

In normal people, positive nitrogen balance shows up at just the right times. Children, pregnant women and convalescents all will have positive nitrogen balances. The body needs extra nitrogen and it takes it.

Most of the time most of us are in proper nitrogen balance. Usually the nitrogen our body consumes is equal to the nitrogen that it gives out as waste. New cells replace old; new nitrogen replaces old. It is as simple as that.

It is important to understand the role of protein in our general health, but if you are obese you can all but forget protein as the cause. We now, I think, are ready to turn to those much maligned substances which work in different ways, which perform different functions, but which are all grouped together under the single word *fat*.

Human fat is different from animal fat, which is different from fish fat, which in turn is different from vegetable fat. Chicken fat is different from all these and even varies from chicken to chicken, depending on the food the bird has eaten.

To begin your comprehension of the role fat plays in our lives, understand first that we need fat to function normally. Here are some of the things fat does:

1. It provides roundness to the body. Although you probably have not thought of fat in relation to beauty, fat is very important to the body of a beautiful woman. A woman with an ideal figure has an ideal distribution of body fat.

2. It keeps the skin soft and supple. Fat under the skin and fat working among the cells of the skin itself provide for good complexion and good skin tone.

3. It gives your body energy. Fat, as you know, burns clean and hot. As it burns, you get energy.

4. Fat helps promote normal growth. Through com-

121

plicated body processes, fat helps conserve important proteins, while carbohydrates tend to rob the body of proteins. People whose diet lacks sufficient fat are undersized.

5. Fat influences digestion and the absorption of other foodstuffs in your system. Without sufficient fat, you don't get what you should out of the other food substances you eat.

6. Fat affects the rate at which your bones calcify. Calcium is a major element in the bones and calcification is the process by which bones harden and by which broken bones are repaired. Without sufficient fat, calcification is impeded.

7. Fat helps transport certain essential vitamins through the body. These vitamins are fat-soluble, which is to say they dissolve in fat. Fat is the vehicle in which these vitamins travel to key points in the body, just as a river may be a vehicle in transporting certain elements to the sea.

8. Fat, the right kind of fat, controls your weight. You need to eat fat if you are to be slim.

Human body fat is an oily liquid that is stored in a mass of cells in the delicate adipose (fatty) tissue, much as honey is stored in a honeycomb. Adipose tissue covers most of your body and is also found in certain internal organs. The chemical components from which human fat is formed are called triglycerides, and these triglycerides are made up of certain acids. Human fat is different from animal fats in that it contains different percentages

122

of triglycerides. The fat of a horse or a wild rabbit contains linolenic acid. There is no linolenic acid found in human fat. (I suspect that the horse and the wild rabbit derive the linolenic acid from grass.)

The triglycerides of animal fat are referred to as "saturated" fat, while the fat found in marine life contains a large amount of "unsaturated" fat. What is the difference? It involves a little chemistry, but this is chemistry well worth knowing. For it is just this chemistry that will explain why you can lose weight on a high-fat diet. This diet will be rich in the *unsaturated* fatty acids.

The term "saturated" is not used in the sense with which you are familiar. It refers to the character of the molecules which make up fats. As you may remember from high-school chemistry, molecules are infinitesimal particles of substance. A molecule is the smallest physical unit of an element or of a compound.

Molecules, of course, are capable of joining with other molecules. A slab of steel represents millions and millions of molecules tightly joined together. The way molecules link up with one another is one of the basic studies of chemistry.

In a saturated fat, chemically speaking, the molecule of carbon joins in a single link with the contiguous molecule of carbon. But in an unsaturated fatty acid, the carbon molecule is not so congenial; it will link up with another molecule of carbon, but it requires a double link. When there are several chains of double-linked carbon molecules in a fat, the fat is called "polyunsaturated" (from the Greek *poly* meaning "several"). These polyunsaturated fatty acids have recently been recognized as of vital importance in human nutrition. There are also monounsaturated fatty acids, fats which contain in their chain only one double link. Olive oil is very rich in them. Monounsaturated fatty acids are of a neutral nature and neither increase nor decrease the level of cholesterol in the blood. Saturated fats raise the cholesterol level, while polyunsaturated fats lower it.

Probably you have heard the term "polyunsaturated" before. It appears, quite properly, on the labels of several commercially marketed vegetable oils. A television advertising campaign for one such oil stressed that it was "polyunsaturated." This was good for you, the announcer explained, and he let it go at that. The commercial was short, which may have been one reason. Then, too, a good deal of advertising is based on the fact that many people accept things on faith. If enough people hear that something is good for them enough times, some will believe it without knowing quite why.

In a sense, it was unfortunate that polyunsaturated fatty acids were plugged as "good for you," just as foolish formulas for losing weight are plugged as "harmless." It is unfortunate because polyunsaturated fatty acids are indeed good for you, even though they have been plugged on television. So if you are one of those naturally skeptical people who doubt all advertising claims, I ask you, in this one case, to lay aside your skepticism. Even though the announcer may not have known why, polyunsaturated fatty acids are every bit as valuable as he claimed.

We can return to the fatty acids after we consider how your body forms its fat. As we know, body fat is created from food, largely from carbohydrates. In a lean person who is maintaining his weight, the carbohydrates are broken down to create energy and just enough fat to sustain the proper level—11 per cent of body weight. But if things are not working smoothly, we run into that pyruvic-acid difficulty. No one yet knows precisely why an obese person cannot properly handle the pyruvic acid that comes from carbohydrates. Perhaps the difficulty stems from an insufficient production of enzymes, those substances which enable us to digest our food. Perhaps it is some other complication. As I say, no one yet knows, but we do know that in 95 per cent of all obese people normal metabolism stops at the level of pyruvic acid.

Instead of smoothly converting this acid to energy, carbon dioxide and water, the obese person's system stalls. Ultimately the pyruvic acid becomes triglycerides, which presently are deposited about the body as fat. The liver is involved in this, and so is fat tissue itself. For fat tissue, which scientists long believed was inert, has now been demonstrated to have an active life of its own. Fat tissue can create more fat from carbohydrates, it can regulate where the new fat is deposited, and it can control the rate at which new fat is absorbed by old.

The problems in controlling weight, then, are twofold: We want first to control the problem of pyruvic acid, something we can achieve by limiting carbohydrates. Then we want to control the character of the fat itself. This, as you'll see, can be achieved by a diet rich in the polyunsaturated fatty acids. For the most part, these are contained in fish and in vegetable oils, rather than in meat. Vegetable oils play a vital role in my new nutrition principle.

A few decades ago scientists believed that all fats were burned by the body until the body had derived sufficient energy from them, and that then the excess, and only the excess, was distributed through the body in the form of fat deposits. Today we know otherwise. Body fat is the result of carbohydrate synthesis. Dietetic fat is burned almost in entirety. As Pennington has proven, the human body has unlimited capacity to burn fats.

Scientists also once believed that fat was inert storage material. Since we know that fat produces more fat, we know this is not so. Fat is constantly involved in the metabolic process. Further, your fat itself is subject to change. In one experiment scientists fed hogs large quantities of liquid fats. The lard on these animal's bodies became softer. Then, when the hogs were switched back to diets high in carbohydrates, the lard on their bodies again became hard and tough. If you assume from this that the first step in a human's losing excess fat is the softening of the fat itself, you are correct. But you are getting ahead of the story.

In research on the nature of fat in the body, scientists have discovered other things that would have startled the medical men of earlier times. For one thing, we know now that the burning of fat provides us with at least 60 per cent of our energy. Carbohydrates, which were once thought to provide most of our energy, actually serve chiefly to help make the fat we need for energy. And there are better ways to take in the elements of fat than by eating carbohydrates. For another thing, we know that all fatty acids are not the same. Scientists once believed that all these substances, which both form fats and provide the body with energy, were virtually identical. But it has been discovered that certain specific fatty acids are unique and essential to nutrition. They cannot be skipped; the body will accept no substitutes. The original experiments were done on rats in a laboratory. The rats, not fed the necessary fatty acids, but given a diet complete in protein, carbohydrate, vitamins and minerals, developed scaly skin and kidney damage, and ultimately they died. From this the scientists concluded:

1. Certain specific fatty acids are vital to health.

2. The body cannot create them itself. It must take them in with food.

Since these fatty acids are essential to health, they have been labeled "essential fatty acids." Many American diets are deficient in them. Remember, they are unsaturated—the kind of fat we get from fish and from vegetable oils, but *do not* get from meat. Only in the last few years has the role of the essential fatty acids in controlling obesity become clear. But earlier scientists had learned the important role of these substances in other areas of health. Here are some of them:

1. Numerous skin conditions seem to occur when the

body does not get enough of the essential fatty acids. Working with animals, investigators have been able to cause and cure a great number of skin disorders by with-holding, then administering, the essential fatty acids. Among humans, investigators have discovered that a deficiency in the essential fatty acids increases the susceptibility of the skin to a number of unsightly conditions. Some investigators have found them to be helpful in clearing or easing eczema.

In a study of 20,000 infants, skin disorders were found to occur seven times more frequently in bottle-fed than in breast-fed babies. (Mother's milk contains considerably more of the essential fatty acids than does cow's milk.) Recently one leading manufacturer of evaporated milk, a product used in preparing infants' formulas, removed a great amount of animal fat and replaced it with corn oil, a substance rich in essential fatty acids. It is reported that the incidence of skin disorders is considerably lower than average among the infants fed with corn-oil milk.

If you are obese and have a skin condition, such as scaly hands or poor complexion, a deficiency in essential fatty acids is probably to blame, at least in part.

2. Sinus trouble and susceptibility to colds both seem to be helped in some cases by essential fatty acids. The body handles these substances easily. It appears to be easier for a body to maintain the proper level of moisture in the mucous membranes when the diet contains a sufficient amount of essential fatty acids.

3. Cholesterol level in the blood is lowered by unsatu-

128

rated fatty acids. In the chapter on the ills that come with obesity, we considered the influence of cholesterol in diseases of the blood vessels, in high blood pressure and in coronary attacks. Most scientists believe that a high level of cholesterol contributes to these grave afflictions, and some believe that it is the major cause.

Most animal fats raise cholesterol levels, but the unsaturated fatty acids in vegetable and fish oils work the other way, even in the case of people who have previously suffered from heart seizures and who have histories of high cholesterol levels. The evidence, then, is that people, whether victims of obesity or not, who maintain an abnormally high cholesterol level, do well to include highly unsaturated vegetable oils in their diet.

Hardening of the arteries is a condition which we believe is often caused by an excess of cholesterol in the blood stream. Experiments have demonstrated that unsaturated fatty acids both help prevent hardening of the arteries from developing and improve existing conditions, even of long standing. The unsaturated fatty acids work effectively even when the rest of the diet is high in cholesterol. An incidental, but important, point is that a fat-free diet, necessarily high in carbohydrates, raises the cholesterol level in the blood.

These considerations are important, but, laying them aside, we come to the question of unsaturated fatty acids and obesity. This is our basic question. By now you can understand why carbohydrates make you fat and why you must sharply limit the amount of sugar and starch you allow yourself to eat. But what about fat? You *must* eat fat to lose fat, and you *must* eat a good deal of unsaturated fat, probably far more than you have been eating. Some of the reasons are simple; some are more involved. Let's consider the simple one first.

Fat lengthens the digestive process. You digest fat more slowly than you digest carbohydrates and so you do not get hungry soon after eating fat. This is appetite inhibiting in its proper sense. By eating fat you are following the natural way to appetite control. Then, too, fat provides you with concentrated energy. What you eat you digest slowly. Since there is a steady, intense flow of energy, you are less likely to suffer an energy lag between meals. After you adjust to a diet rich in unsaturated fats, you will probably find that the need for snacks between meals will disappear. In most cases, it does.

These points show how unsaturated fats help control weight *gain*. Now we can proceed to see how they work to rid your body of excess fat that has been on your frame for years.

We know obesity is caused by two conditions. The first is called excessive lipogenesis: excessive formation of fat. (*Genesis* comes from the Greek word for origin.) The second is decreased lipolysis: insufficient breaking down of fat. (*Lysis*, another word from the Greek, refers to a breaking down.)

By cutting down on carbohydrates, we are working to control the formation of fat within the body. By increasing the fat intake—specifically, the intake of unsaturated fats—we are increasing the breaking down of fat within the body. We are squeezing the excess body fat in two ways; we are squeezing it out of your system.

When you eat large quantities of unsaturated fats, you set in motion a happy cycle. You *stimulate* body production of certain hormones which work to release fats stored around the body. You *limit* the production of insulin, a substance which seems to prevent the release of stored fat. And you change the character of your fat. The hard, tough fat, difficult for the body to utilize, softens.

In essence, I have demonstrated this by analyzing the fat in patients' blood. We all have fatty substances in our blood stream, but for many years it was assumed that fat was fat, just as it was assumed that calories were calories. Actually, there are different types of fat in the blood stream, and what a researcher now must do is "fraction" the fat. He must check the different types of fat that are present and measure each one individually instead of measuring these fats as though they were a single unit.

When the body is storing and depositing a great deal of fat, the blood stream is overburdened with triglycerides. The blood stream, like a river, carries the triglycerides about the body. Then it drops them off at your midsection or at your neck, where existing fat helps turn the triglycerides into bulges.

When the body is taking stored fat from the bulges and burning it through the liver, the blood stream is rich in phospholipids. The blood stream, again acting like a river, carries the excess fat from the bulging portions of

131

the body in the form of these phospholipids. At the liver the phospholipids are broken down further, and eventually they are spilled in the urine as fat particles, or ketones.

This balance between triglycerides (fat going to be deposited) and phospholipids (fat coming back to be disposed of in urine) is an amazingly precise measure. From it I can tell how fast a patient is likely to have been gaining weight, how fast a patient under treatment is losing weight, and whether or not a patient has been adhering closely to the principle.

When you limit your intake of carbohydrates, you keep the level of triglycerides low. You don't store new fat. To get the existing fat out of your body, to raise your phospholipid level, you must eat fat. But if you eat just any fat, you run the risk of increasing your cholesterol level. So the one safe way to rid yourself of existing body fat is to make your diet rich in unsaturated fats. These unsaturated fats bring up the phospholipid level. They soften your body fat and help get it out of your system. But at the same time they keep your cholesterol level down. With these unsaturated fats you eat a high-fat diet in absolute safety. The unsaturated fats help you to reduce *and* rid your body of cholesterol, one substance that seems to make heart disease more likely. Used properly, these unsaturated fats are a perfect food.

Under the new nutrition principle you eat unlimited amounts of unsaturated fats, *regardless of their calorie content*. You limit your intake of saturated fats—chiefly animal fats—not because of their calorie content but to keep your cholesterol down. You eat a good deal of protein. The one thing you sharply limit is carbohydrate, which is to say bread, many fruits and vegetables, and other foods, which are all mentioned in the next chapter.

On this program you will not lose all your extra fat in a week, but you will lose steadily—as steadily as your body can safely rid itself of long-stored fat. No "diet" is regulating your loss of fat; your body is regulating itself. It is being encouraged to lose fat naturally, and it will respond. Your body may, and almost certainly will, respond differently from your neighbor's. No two individuals are the same. Whatever rate of fat loss your body assumes on a diet that is comfortable to you—on a diet rich in fats that does not produce nausea—is the proper rate. The whole process may take six months or a year, but be patient with your body and the process will be successful and complete.

When you have lost all your extra fat, when your body is about 11 per cent fat, you will stop losing weight. Again, the body will be regulating itself. (I might mention that lean people following my nutrition principle do not lose; only excess fat is affected.)

With these points understood, I think you are ready to turn to specifics. We can now consider just what rules to follow, just what foods to eat, just what changes you may want to make in your kitchen. In short, we are ready to turn from theory to practice.

# CHAPTER EIGHT

# YOUR "DIET"

IF YOU CAME TO MY OFFICE in order to lose weight, we would begin with a discussion of your eating habits. I would ask questions to find out just how long you have been obese, how heavily you have gone in for carbohydrates, if emotional problems have contributed toward your obesity, if you have the symptoms of any disease. I would take a small blood sample from you and, of course, give you a complete physical examination.

We cannot do all of that here, but I can provide you with some questions to ask yourself. When you have answered them, you will better understand the individual difficulties connected with your individual case of obesity.

Here, to begin, is a food table which tells you just what foods are rich in carbohydrate, what foods are rich in protein and what foods are rich in fat. On the extreme left I list the name of the food. The next column tells you how much of the food makes up a 100-gram portion. Then, in the final columns, headed "Proportions" I give you the amount of carbohydrates, proteins and fats that such a portion of each food contains. The letter $C$ stands for "carbohydrate," the letter $P$ stands for "protein," and the letter $F$ stands for "fat." *Gm.*, of course, stands for "gram."

134

The table is here for you to read and to study. It is a quick reference you can use in preparing your daily menu. But you can use it also as a measure of your calorie intake. As the table indicates, a gram of carbohydrate or of protein provides you with four calories, while a gram of fat provides you with nine calories. When you adjust your diet to my new nutrition principle you will see how your fat vanishes while you are taking in many thousands of calories a day. Remember, then, that you want to concentrate on foods in which the carbohydrate content is low—regardless of the total calorie count.

## FOOD TABLE

*Showing amounts of carbohydrate, protein and fat present in 100-gm. portions of common foods*

### I. CEREALS, BREAD, AND OTHER FLOUR PRODUCTS

| | 100-Gm. Portion (Household Measure) | Proportions (in Grams)* | | |
| --- | --- | --- | --- | --- |
| | | C | P | F |
| Bread: white, rye or whole wheat | 3½ slices (½" thick) | 50 | 9 | 3 |
| Cake or cookies (without fruit or icing) | 1 slice (3"x3"x1½") | 65 | 6 | 9 |
| Cereal: whole wheat, rice, rye or oat | | 77 | 11 | 1 |
| Crackers, Graham | 10 to 12 large | 72 | 9 | 9 |
| Crackers, matzoth | | 70 | 15 | 0 |
| Crackers, soda | 25 (2"x2") | 73 | 10 | 9 |
| Doughnuts | 2 | 52 | 7 | 22 |
| Hominy, cooked | ½ cup | 15 | 2 | 0 |
| Macaroni, cooked | ⅔ cup | 18 | 3 | 0 |

# I. CEREALS, BREAD, AND OTHER FLOUR PRODUCTS (Continued)

| | 100-Gm. Portion (Household Measure) | Proportions (in Grams)* | | |
|---|---|---|---|---|
| | | C | P | F |
| Macaroni, raw | ¾ cup | 74 | 13 | 1 |
| Noodles, cooked | ½ cup | 20 | 4 | 0 |
| Rice | ½ cup | 24 | 3 | 0 |
| Spaghetti, cooked | ½ cup | 20 | 4 | 0 |

*1 gram C or P = 4 calories; 1 gram F = 9 calories.

# II. DAIRY PRODUCTS

| | 100-Gm. Household Portion | Proportions (in Grams) | | |
|---|---|---|---|---|
| | | C | P | F |
| Milk, whole | ⅖ cup | 5 | 4 | 4 |
| Milk, skimmed | ⅖ cup | 5 | 4 | 0 |
| Milk, evaporated | ⅖ cup | 10 | 7 | 8 |
| Milk, powdered, skimmed | ¾ cup | 52 | 36 | 1 |
| Milk, malted, dry | ¾ cup | 72 | 15 | 9 |
| Buttermilk | ½ cup | 5 | 4 | 1 |
| Cream, 10% (light) | ⅖ cup | 5 | 4 | 12 |
| Cream, 20% (average) | ⅖ cup | 5 | 3 | 19 |
| Cream, 40% (heavy) | ⅖ cup | 3 | 2 | 41 |
| Ice Cream (without fruit or nuts) | ½ cup | 20 | 4 | 13 |
| Butter (or oleomargarine | 10 square (1″x1″x½″) | 0 | 1 | 81 |
| Cheese, American | 1 slice (4″x2″x1″) | 2 | 27 | 32 |
| Cheese, cottage | 6 level tbsp. | 4 | 20 | 1 |
| Cheese, cream | 5 squares (1″x1″x¾″) | 2 | 7 | 34 |
| Cheese, other | ⅖ cup | 2 | 20 | 32 |

## III. EGGS

| | 100-Gm. Household Portion | Proportions (in Grams) | | |
|---|---|---|---|---|
| | | C | P | F |
| Egg, whole | 1 medium (60 Gm.) | 0 | 6 | 6 |
| Egg White | 1 white only | 0 | 3 | 0 |
| Egg Yolk | 1 yolk only | 0 | 3 | 6 |

## IV. FISH (RAW, UNLESS OTHER-WISE SPECIFIED)

| | 100-Gm. Household Portion | Proportions (in Grams) | | |
|---|---|---|---|---|
| | | C | P | F |
| Bass | 2 slices (4″x2″x½″) | 0 | 20 | 2 |
| Clams, meat only | ½ cup | 5 | 11 | 1 |
| Cod | 2 slices (4″x2″x½″) | 0 | 20 | 1 |
| Crabmeat, canned | ⅔ cup | 1 | 17 | 3 |
| Fish, other | ⅔ cup | 0 | 19 | 8 |
| Halibut | 2 slices (4″x2″x½″) | 0 | 18 | 6 |
| Herring | ½ medium fish | 0 | 20 | 7 |
| Herring, smoked | ½ medium fish | 0 | 37 | 16 |
| Lobster, fresh or canned | ¾ cup | 0 | 18 | 1 |
| Oysters, meat only | 4 or 5 large | 5 | 8 | 1 |
| Salmon, fresh or canned | ¾ cup | 0 | 21 | 12 |
| Sardines, canned | 4 large or 10 small | 0 | 23 | 20 |
| Scallops | ½ cup | 3 | 15 | 0 |
| Shrimp | ½ cup | 1 | 18 | 1 |

# V. FRUITS
## GROUP 1 (APPROXIMATELY 5% C)

| | 100-Gm. Household Portion | Proportions (in Grams) | | |
|---|---|---|---|---|
| | | C | P | F |
| Avocado | ½, 4″ long | 3 | 2 | 26 |
| Muskmelon (cantaloupe or honeydew) | ¼ melon (5″ diam.) | 5 | 1 | 0 |
| Watermelon (edible portion) | 1 slice (2″x2″x2″) | 6 | 0 | 0 |

## GROUP 2 (APPROXIMATELY 10% C)

| | | C | P | F |
|---|---|---|---|---|
| Blackberries | ½ cup | 8 | 11 | 1 |
| Cranberries | ¼ cup (cooked) | 10 | 1 | 1 |
| Currants | ½ cup | 10 | 2 | 0 |
| Gooseberries | ⅔ cup | 8 | 1 | 0 |
| Grapefruit | ½ (4″ diam.) or ⅖ cup juice | 10 | 0 | 0 |
| Lemon | 1 (2½″ long) or ½ cup juice | 8 | 1 | 0 |
| Papaya | ¼ (5″ diam.) | 9 | 1 | 0 |
| Tangerine | 2 small or ½ cup juice | 9 | 1 | 0 |

## GROUP 3 (APPROXIMATELY 15% C)

| | | C | P | F |
|---|---|---|---|---|
| Apple | 1 small (¾ medium) | 14 | 0 | 0 |
| Apple juice | ½ cup | 13 | 0 | 0 |
| Applesauce | ½ cup | 13 | 0 | 0 |
| Apricots (fresh) | 1½ average | 13 | 1 | 0 |
| Blueberries | ⅔ cup or ⅔ cup juice | 15 | 1 | 1 |
| Grapes | ¾ cup | 15 | 1 | 1 |
| Huckleberries | ⅔ cup or ⅖ cup juice | 14 | 0 | 0 |

138

# V. FRUITS (Continued)

## GROUP 3 (APPROXIMATELY 15% C)

|  | 100-Gm. Household Portion | Proportions (in Grams) | | |
|---|---|---|---|---|
|  |  | C | P | F |
| Limes | 1 (2½″ long) | 13 | 0 | 0 |
| Loganberries | ⅔ cup | 14 | 1 | 1 |
| Mulberries | ⅔ cup | 13 | 0 | 0 |
| Nectarines | 2 medium | 14 | 0 | 0 |
| Orange | 1 medium or ⅖ cup juice | 13 | 0 | 0 |
| Peaches | 1 medium (2½″) | 12 | 1 | 0 |
| Pears | 1 medium | 14 | 1 | 0 |
| Pineapple, fresh or canned | ⅔ cup or 1 slice 3″ thick | 14 | 0 | 0 |
| Pineapple juice | ½ cup | 14 | 0 | 0 |
| Plums, fresh | 3 (1½″ diam.) | 12 | 1 | 0 |
| Quince, fresh | ⅓ (2½″x3″) | 12 | 0 | 0 |
| Raspberries | ⅔ cup or ½ cup juice | 12 | 1 | 1 |

## GROUP 4 (APPROXIMATELY 20% C)

| Banana | 1 medium, ½ large | 22 | 1 | 0 |
|---|---|---|---|---|
| Cherries | ⅔ cup | 17 | 1 | 1 |
| Figs, fresh | 2 medium (1½″) | 18 | 1 | 0 |
| Grape juice | ½ cup | 19 | 0 | 0 |
| Persimmons, Japanese | 1 large | 18 | 1 | 0 |
| Prune juice (canned) | ½ glass | 18 | 0 | 0 |
| Prunes, fresh | 3 to 4 | 19 | 1 | 0 |

## GROUP 5 (ABOVE 20% C)

| Cherries, Maraschino | ½ cup | 50 | 0 | 0 |
|---|---|---|---|---|
| Currants, dried | ½ cup | 70 | 2 | 0 |
| Dates, fresh | 18 medium | 65 | 2 | 0 |
| Dates, dry | 14 medium | 78 | 2 | 3 |

139

# V. FRUITS (Continued)
## GROUP 5 (ABOVE 20% C)

|  | 100-Gm. Household Portion | Proportions (in Grams) | | |
|---|---|---|---|---|
|  |  | C | P | F |
| Figs, dry | 8 to 10 | 68 | 4 | 0 |
| Persimmons, native, fresh | 2 small | 28 | 1 | 0 |
| Prunes, dried | 10 medium | 65 | 2 | 0 |
| Raisins, dried | ⅔ cup | 75 | 3 | 3 |

# VI. MEAT AND POULTRY (RAW, UNLESS OTHERWISE SPECIFIED)

|  | 100-Gm. Household Portion | Proportions (in Grams) | | |
|---|---|---|---|---|
|  |  | C | P | F |
| Bacon | 10 slices (2″x4″x⅛″) | 0 | 9 | 65 |
| Bacon, crisp | 20 slices (2″x3″x⅛″) | 0 | 30 | 50 |
| Beef, medium fat, medium roasted | 2 slices (2″x3″x1″) | 0 | 20 | 11 |
| Beef, lean, broiled | 2 slices (2″x3″x1″) | 0 | 28 | 5 |
| Beef, fat, medium done | 2 slices (2″x3″x1″) | 0 | 13 | 18 |
| Chicken or duck |  | 0 | 21 | 5 |
| Frankfurter (all meat) | 2 average size | 1 | 19 | 18 |
| Ham, fresh, lean | 2 slices (2″x2″x½″) | 0 | 25 | 14 |
| Ham, fresh, fat | 2 slices (4″x3″x½″) | 0 | 12 | 40 |
| Heart, beef | 2 slices (2″x3″x½″) | 0 | 16 | 20 |
| Heart, pork | 1 slice (2″x3″x1″) | 0 | 17 | 6 |
| Kidney | ½ cup | 0 | 16 | 6 |
| Lamb (or mutton) | 2 slices (1″x4″x1″) | 0 | 19 | 15 |

## VI. MEAT AND POULTRY (RAW, UNLESS OTHERWISE SPECIFIED) (Continued)

| | 100-Gm. Household Portion | Proportions (in Grams) | | |
|---|---|---|---|---|
| | | C | P | F |
| Lamb (or mutton) chops | 2 chops | 0 | 20 | 22 |
| Liver | 2 slices (3"x2"x½") | 0 | 20 | 5 |
| Pork, lean | 1 slice (2"x3"x3") | 0 | 16 | 24 |
| Sausage (all meat) | 6 (3"x¾") | 0 | 18 | 38 |
| Tongue | 5 slices (¼" thick) | 0 | 16 | 15 |
| Turkey | 2 slices (4"x3"x½") | 0 | 22 | 18 |
| Veal, medium fat | 2 slices (2"x3"x½") | 0 | 20 | 8 |

## VII. VEGETABLES

### GROUP 1 (APPROXIMATELY 5% CARBOHYDRATE)

| | 100-Gm. Household Portion | Proportions (in Grams) | | |
|---|---|---|---|---|
| | | C | P | F |
| Artichokes (French) | 1 medium | 3 | 1 | 0 |
| Asparagus | ½ cup tips or 10 stalks | 3 | 1 | 0 |
| Beans, string | ¾ cup | 3 | 1 | 0 |
| Beet greens | ½ cup | 4 | 2 | 0 |
| Broccoli | ⅔ cup | 4 | 3 | 0 |
| Brussels sprouts | 10 sprouts | 4 | 1 | 0 |
| Cabbage | ⅔ to 1 cup | 4 | 1 | 0 |
| Cauliflower | ⅔ cup | 2 | 1 | 0 |
| Celery | 2 hearts or 4 stalks | 3 | 1 | 0 |
| Chard leaves | 2 to 3 cups | 4 | 3 | 0 |
| Cucumber | ½ cup | 2 | 1 | 0 |

141

## VII. VEGETABLES (Continued)

### GROUP 1 (APPROXIMATELY 5% CARBOHYDRATE) (Continued)

| | 100-Gm. Household Portion | Proportions (in Grams) C | P | F |
|---|---|---|---|---|
| Eggplant | ¾ cup | 4 | 1 | 0 |
| Endive | 2 small | 2 | 1 | 0 |
| Escarole | ⅔ small head | 2 | 1 | 0 |
| Kale | ⅔ cup | 5 | 2 | 0 |
| Leek | ¾ cup | 5 | 2 | 0 |
| Lettuce | ⅓ small head | 2 | 1 | 0 |
| Mushrooms | ½ cup | 1 | 1 | 0 |
| Okra | ½ cup | 4 | 1 | 0 |
| Peppers, green | 1 medium (3″ to 4″ long) | 4 | 1 | 0 |
| Pumpkin | ½ cup | 6 | 1 | 0 |
| Radishes | 10 medium | 3 | 1 | 0 |
| Rhubarb | ⅔ cup | 3 | 1 | 0 |
| Sauerkraut | ⅔ cup | 3 | 1 | 0 |
| Spinach | ½ cup | 2 | 1 | 0 |
| Squash, summer | ⅔ cup | 3 | 1 | 0 |
| Tomatoes | 1 medium or ½ cup | 4 | 1 | 0 |
| Turnip (beet or greens) | ½ cup | 5 | 1 | 0 |
| Watercress | 1 medium bunch | 2 | 1 | 0 |

### GROUP 2 (APPROXIMATELY 10% C)

| | | C | P | F |
|---|---|---|---|---|
| Beans, dry soy | ½ cup | 7 | 35 | 18 |
| Beet root | ½ cup | 9 | 2 | 0 |
| Carrots | ⅔ cup | 8 | 1 | 0 |
| Dandelion greens | ½ cup (cooked) | 7 | 3 | 1 |
| Onion, white | ½ cup (5 or 6 small) | 9 | 2 | 0 |
| Peas, green (fresh or canned) | ½ cup | 9 | 4 | 0 |

142

## VII. VEGETABLES (Continued)

### GROUP 2 (APPROXIMATELY 10% C) (Cont.)

|  | 100-Gm. Household Portion | Proportions (in Grams) | | |
|---|---|---|---|---|
|  |  | C | P | F |
| Peppers, red | 1 medium (3″ to 4″ long) | 7 | 1 | 1 |
| Rutabaga | ⅔ cup | 7 | 1 | 0 |
| Squash, winter | ¾ cup | 7 | 1 | 0 |

### GROUP 3 (APPROXIMATELY 15% C)

|  |  | | | |
|---|---|---|---|---|
| Beans, lima | ½ cup | 15 | 4 | 0 |
| Parsnips | ½ cup | 16 | 2 | 1 |

### GROUP 4 (APPROXIMATELY 20% C)

|  |  | | | |
|---|---|---|---|---|
| Beans, baked, canned | ½ cup | 19 | 6 | 2 |
| Beans, dry | ½ cup | 62 | 22 | 2 |
| Beans, kidney, canned | ½ cup | 17 | 7 | 0 |
| Chili sauce | ⅓ cup | 20 | 0 | 0 |
| Corn | ⅓ cup | 19 | 3 | 1 |
| Lentils | ½ cup | 57 | 25 | 1 |
| Potato | 1 medium (2½″ diam.) | 19 | 2 | 1 |
| Potato chips | 4 cups | 49 | 7 | 37 |
| Potato, sweet | 1 small or ½ medium | 26 | 3 | 0 |
| Succotash, canned | ⅔ cup | 18 | 4 | 1 |

## VIII. MISCELLANEOUS FOODS

|  | 100-Gm. Household Portion | Proportions (in Grams) | | |
|---|---|---|---|---|
|  |  | C | P | F |
| Beer | ⅖ glass | 4 | 0 | 0 |
| Broth, clear | ½ cup | 0 | 0 | 0 |
| Carbonated drinks | ⅖ glass | 8 to 16 | 0 | 0 |

# VIII. MISCELLANEOUS FOODS
## (Continued)

| | 100-Gm. Household Portion | Proportions (in Grams) | | |
|---|---|---|---|---|
| | | C | P | F |
| Catsup | ⅖ cup | 24 | 2 | 0 |
| Chocolate, sweet, dry | ⅖ cup | 60 | 2 | 25 |
| Chocolate, un-sweetened dry | ⅖ cup | 25 | 12 | 52 |
| Cocoa, dry, un-sweetened | ¾ cup | 38 | 18 | 20 |
| Coconut, prepared | 1 cup | 52 | 4 | 39 |
| Cod liver oil | ⅖ cup | 0 | 0 | 0 |
| Custard | ½ cup | 5 | 6 | 7 |
| Dextrose | ⅖ cup | 100 | 0 | 0 |
| Fat, cooking | ⅖ cup | 0 | 0 | 100 |
| Flour | 1½ cups | 76 | 11 | 1 |
| Gelatin, dry | ⅔ cup | 0 | 85 | 0 |
| Honey | ⅓ cup | 81 | 0 | 0 |
| Jelly | ⅓ cup | 70 | 0 | 0 |
| Lard (or other shortening) | ⅖ cup | 0 | 0 | 100 |
| Marmalade | ⅓ cup | 65 | 1 | 0 |
| Mayonnaise | ⅖ cup | 0 | 2 | 75 |
| Molasses | ½ cup | 60 | 0 | 0 |
| Nuts, miscellaneous (meats) | | 20 | 2 | 60 |
| Oils, salad and cook-ing | ⅖ cup | 0 | 0 | 100 |
| Olives, ripe or green | 18 | 3 | 2 | 15 |
| Pickles, sour | ⅓ cup | 2 | 0.5 | 0 |
| Pickles, sweet, mixed | 1 cup | 25 | 1 | 0 |
| Popcorn, popped | 6 cups | 80 | 12 | 5 |
| Salad dressing | ⅓ cup | 15 | 5 | 10 |
| Soup, commercial, undiluted (see labels) | ⅖ cup | 10 | 3 | 2 |

# VIII. MISCELLANEOUS FOODS
## (Continued)

| | 100-Gm. Household Portion | Proportions (in Grams) | | |
|---|---|---|---|---|
| | | C | P | F |
| Soup, creamed | ½ cup | 4 | 2 | 13 |
| Soybean, dry | ½ cup | 12 | 34 | 18 |
| Soybean, fresh | ⅔ cup | 6 | 13 | 7 |
| Starch, corn | ¾ cup | 87 | 1 | 0 |
| Sugar, granulated | ⅖ cup | 100 | 0 | 0 |
| Tapioca pudding | ⅔ cup | 28 | 3 | 3 |
| Vinegar | ⅖ cup | 4 | 0 | 0 |
| Yeast | 100 Gm. | 8 | 8 | 0 |

Here are some questions I will ask in establishing a nutrition pattern that is ideal for you. You now should ask them of yourself.

1. What did you have for breakfast today? Lunch? Dinner? (When you ask yourself this, check to see if your meals were rich in carbohydrates.)

2. What snacks did you eat between meals?

3. Do you eat much cake? Candy?

4. Do you eat before going to bed?

5. Do you drink? How much?

6. How much exercise do you take in a normal day?

7. Do you crave certain foods? Do you eat compulsively? Do you find yourself eating just to pass the time?

8. How long have you been heavy? Did your weight increase suddenly? Was your life upset just before your weight gain?

9. What have you done previously to lose weight?

From questions of this sort I get a good picture of my patient's eating habits and general health. And from the blood sample I learn two very important factors: how fast the patient is forming fat and how fast the patient is getting rid of fat. (Remember, the triglycerides tell me about fat formation and the phospholipids tell me about the disposal of fat.)

Naturally, with all these checks, I can be very precise in my office. I can say almost to the spoonful how many carbohydrates someone may safely have. Here I must be more general, but, by approaching my new nutrition principle carefully and sensibly, you should be able to achieve excellent results yourself. Begin with these fourteen general rules, your own Fourteen Points:

1. You *must* have three full meals at regular intervals each day; do not leave the table hungry.

2. You do not have to count calories, but do not eat *any* of the foods that are not permitted.

3. The slightest deviation from this program will hold back your weight loss for a considerable time.

4. Make sure that you eat fish or sea food once a day, because marine food is rich in unsaturated fatty acids.

5. Have fried foods every day, frying them in margarine or in the vegetable oils I will list for you. These oils and margarine are both rich in unsaturated fatty acids.

6. Do not skip a meal. Even if you are not hungry, force yourself to eat at least some food containing unsaturated fat.

7. Don't worry about taking in too much fat. Your body will let you know when you have had enough. (The sign of eating too much fat is nausea.)

8. Drink plenty of water—at least three glasses between one meal and the next.

9. Generally avoid dried foodstuffs.

10. Do not add salt to your food.

11. Avoid alcohol. In the beginning it is best if you avoid all alcohol, eliminating even wine with meals.

12. Do not check your weight on a scale. We are

146

treating obesity, not overweight. The fit of your clothing will tell you how successful you are.

    13. Walk at least one hour a day.

    14. Do not eat between meals or within three hours of going to bed.

With these rules in mind, we are ready to move on to further specifics: what to eat and what not to eat. Here are the foods to eat:

    1. All meats (but first trim the visible fat).

    2. All forms of fish and sea food—*with* the natural oils and fats. Preferably, fry the sea food in oils which I shall specify.

    3. All kinds of cheese.

    4. Vegetables, following the table on pages 143–44. That is, eat, in addition to potatoes, only those vegetables that contain no more than 5 per cent carbohydrates. These are listed in Group I. You may have two 3-ounce servings of these vegetables at dinner and at lunch.

    5. Eggs, fried in margarine or a specified oil.

    6. Gluten bread. This is a dietetic product, bread from which most carbohydrate has been removed. Gluten bread is the only permissible form of bread.

    7. Artificially sweetened carbonated soft drinks. These are the drinks without carbohydrate or with only a minute quantity. The label on these drinks will indicate that they are made without carbohydrate.

    8. Coffee and tea. You may add artificial sweeteners, but not sugar.

    9. Shell nuts.

    10. Fruits containing no more than 5 per cent carbohydrate. Again, consult the table to see which fruits these are.

    11. Milk, but not more than a cupful a day. In practice, a little milk with your coffee or tea.

These, then, are the foods you may eat as you begin adopting my new nutrition principle. I think you will agree that it is a wide list. Since it is important for you to eat large quantities of fish and meats, you will not go hungry. In fact, you may have to eat more than you have been eating.

Here are the foods to shun. They must be shunned absolutely. You cannot eat even small amounts of them without greatly impeding your weight loss.

1. Fruits containing more than 5 per cent carbohydrates.
2. Fruit juices of all kinds.
3. Any bread except gluten bread.
4. Sugar and sugar derivatives.
5. Starches of any kind or form.
6. Vegetables rich in carbohydrates.
7. Cakes, cookies or pastries.
8. Candy and chocolate.
9. Ice cream *and* ices.
10. Cream, light or heavy.
11. Carbonated or noncarbonated beverages containing sugar.

How does a typical day's menu look, set up under these instructions? Of course it varies with the skill and imagination of the cook, but here is a sample:

## BREAKFAST

One or two eggs, preferably scrambled in oil or margarine.
One slice of gluten bread with cheese.
Tea or coffee.

## LUNCH

Meat, fowl, fish or sea food. (You must eat at least six to eight ounces.)
Vegetables, chosen as I suggested previously.

One slice of gluten bread.
Tea or coffee.

# DINNER

Meat, fowl, fish or sea food. (At least ten to twelve ounces.)
Vegetables, again following the previous instructions.
One slice of gluten bread.
Tea or coffee.

In addition, you must supplement your diet further in
unsaturated fats. In all, you should take three ounces of
highly unsaturated vegetable oil and eat two ounces of
margarine every day. What kind of margarine? A margarine rich in unsaturated fat. That means, in practice, a
margarine containing corn oil. Not all do. Consult the label
on the package before buying the margarine. Make sure it
contains unsaturated fat.

## OILS CONTAINING UNSATURATED FAT

The key substance in vegetable oils is linoleic acid, an
essential, unsaturated fatty acid. The oils with the greatest quantity of linoleic acid are most valuable in conquering obesity and in keeping cholesterol level low.

| Oil | Percentage of Linoleic Acid |
|---|---|
| Safflower | 75 |
| Corn | 53 |
| Soybean | 50 |
| Cottonseed | 48 |
| Peanut | 25 |
| Olive | 5 |

Clearly, safflower oil is the most valuable by far. This oil, pressed from the seeds of safflowers, is available at most dietetic stores or by order through your grocer. Safflower oil is becoming more easily available, both in liquid form and in capsules obtainable at drug and department stores.

If you cannot obtain safflower oil, corn oil is the next best thing. This oil, pressed, as you can tell, from corn, is on the shelves of supermarkets all across the country. You should have no difficulty in obtaining it. Perhaps you already use it for frying or for salad dressings.

Peanut and olive oil are not helpful for our purposes.

The easiest routine is to take at least two capsules before each meal. There are now capsules of safflower seed oil which contain Vitamin B-6, a valuable factor in the burning of fatty tissue. At least two of these capsules are the required dosage. But individuals with greater excess weight can take proportionally more of the capsules and benefit accordingly. The oils I have listed are your best possible source of unsaturated fatty acids. They represent the best technique yet devised for ridding your body of excess fat while keeping your cholesterol level down. "Have oil, will travel," one of my patients, whose clothing has dropped down two or three sizes, likes to joke. But this is no joke. The oil is essential to the new nutrition principle.

The large portions of meat, fowl or sea food are important, too. It does not matter whether you eat a 6-ounce portion of meat or fish at lunch and a 12-ounce portion at dinner, or whether you prefer to eat the larger portion at midday. The point is that you must eat at least 6 ounces at one meal and at least 10 ounces at the other. What will happen if you do eat less? You will lose weight much more slowly.

Over-all, the average obese person will lose best on a diet which is 65 per cent fat. Two thirds of this fat should be unsaturated. Thirty per cent of the diet should be protein. Only 5 per cent should be carbohydrate.

I think this is a chapter you may want to read several times. You are not likely to memorize the rules of my new nutrition principle in a single reading. But by now several things should be clear. Since you can eat unlimited portions of fish and meat, plus ample helpings of vegetables, you will not go hungry. Since you eat a great deal of fat, your between-meals appetite will be curbed. You have here a program for three sizable meals a day, comprised of the sort of food that digests slowly and will amply supply your body's nutritional needs.

Of course you have questions. All my patients do. (Actually, if you have read carefully, you understand the working of my principle better than most of my patients. There is not time in a physician's crowded day to explain the principle in the great detail that this book has permitted me.)

I think I can anticipate many of your questions. At least I would like to try.

Q: In your office you make analyses of your patients' blood before prescribing an individual diet. How can I be sure the general diet is right for me?

A: Begin with the typical menus I have listed and follow the recipes in the next chapter. If you do not notice definite slimming in a week or two, and physical examination has established that you are not one of the 5 per cent who suffer from grandular obesity, then your carbohydrate metabolism is particularly disturbed. Further cut down your carbohydrate intake. Eliminate the gluten bread. You will then notice a slimming. This principle works because chemistry works. It *cannot fail* to work.

Q: How fast should I expect to lose weight?

A: You should expect to lose fat; consequently you can expect to lose weight.

Q: How fast should I expect to lose fat?

A: The rate varies with the individual. Naturally, the more obese you are, the more dramatically you can lose inches. You did not grow obese overnight, and there is no safe way for you to grow slim in a week or two. Safe slimming is a process of months.

Q: But while I'm losing fat, won't I lose weight too?

A: Unquestionably you will, but not as much as your friends think. Remember, you will be losing fat, a very bulky substance. When you lose 10 pounds of fat you will be considerably slimmer than if, on a low-calorie diet, you had lost 3 pounds of fat and seven of other body substance, such as muscle. When you have lost 10 pounds on this principle, you will be so much slimmer your friends will believe that you have lost 20 or 25.

Q: What about my skin? It's been stretched by fat all these years. Won't it be saggy when I lose inches?

A: Your skin is an amazingly elastic substance. It will

shrink as you shrink. There may be some brief lags, but it will shrink. For extreme cases, certain procedures in plastic surgery are possible. I have never had to recommend them in my practice.

Q: If I drink more than 3 ounces of oil a day, will it hasten my slimming program?

A: It may, but remember, if you want to drink 4 ounces daily, continue to distribute the oil equally among your three meals. As long as you do not feel nausea, you are not giving your body more oil than it can handle.

Q: I'm used to having a snack—cake or ice cream—at three o'clock every afternoon. I don't know if I can simply cut that out.

A: You don't have to readjust completely overnight. Continue the snack for a while, but substitute a piece of cheese or a slice of cold chicken for the cake. And don't test your will power. Simply don't keep cake in the house. When your body adjusts to your new regimen, your hunger between meals will vanish. Usually this is only a matter of a week or so.

Q: But my body needs sweets. I get a certain hunger that only sweets satisfy.

A: Your body does not need sweets. You are used to sweets, which is quite different. You must break yourself of the sweets habit, and, since fat digests slowly, under this program you will find the habit easier to break than you suppose.

Q: Won't my body react violently to such a radical change in my eating habits?

A: Your body will react well. For the first day or two you may feel minor upsets, probably psychological. By the end of a week, these upsets will have vanished.

Q: What about vitamin pills?

A: If you are now taking vitamin pills at the suggestion of your doctor, continue to do so.

Q: Won't I ever be able to drink a martini again?

A: You may. You almost certainly will. After your body has started to slim, try a very dry martini before dinner. Then see what happens. If the slimming stops, then you'd better skip martinis until you've grown still slimmer. If it continues, you will know that the single martini is not doing any damage. However, do not push your luck. Three martinis certainly will do damage to someone with a disturbed carbohydrate metabolism.

Q: Won't I ever be able to eat a piece of candy again?

A: Probably not, but again each individual case is different. If you want to keep an exact check on your fat loss, use a tape measure. Once a week, or every two weeks, measure your neck, chest, waist, hips, thighs and upper arms. By the time you reach the average weights listed in the chart on page 43, your measurements will probably be just right for you. It's at this point that you can experiment cautiously with increasing your carbohydrate intake. But as you do, continue to measure yourself. When the measurements start going up, you have exceeded the amount of carbohydrate that your body can properly handle.

Q: Will the diet make me constipated?

A: If it does, ask your physician to prescribe a bowel softener. The one change sure in your elimination pattern will be an increased output of urine. This is because your body will be ridding itself of stored fats through substances in your urine.

Q: Will the diet have any beneficial effects aside from getting rid of fat?

A: Your general disposition and outlook may improve, because you are nourishing your body properly. Your complexion may improve. You will be less likely to suffer from heartburn. You may experience an increased sexual drive. (These improvements have all been reported to me by many of my patients.)

Q: How will I be able to afford all the new clothes I'll have to buy when I'm slim?

A: I'm afraid that's your problem, but when you encounter it I'm sure you'll find it's a problem you're glad to take on.

This, in a sense, is your reference chapter, one to keep reviewing and to keep studying, for it tells you how to put my new nutrition principle into practice. Once you do, you will start losing excess fat in a way that may surpass your greatest hopes. This has been the history of almost everyone who has adopted the principle and followed it faithfully.

# CHAPTER NINE

# RECIPES TO
# MAKE YOU SLIM

MOST OF THE old nutrition books included sections called "a sample week's menu." I have given you, as I give my patients, a sample day's menu, the better to make clear the new nutrition principle. But I draw a line there. The reason, I suspect, that old "diet" books offered sample menus for a week was that their authors sensed that a week was about as long as the average person could maintain the diet.

My principle outlines a dietary program for the rest of your life. The variety and flavor of your foods will depend, as with all cookery, on ingenuity in the kitchen.

Certain general points are probably already clear to you. Do your frying in oil or in margarine. What you choose in each case is a matter of taste. For anything in which you need bread crumbs, use gluten bread. (Many grocers carry gluten bread; others do not. If your grocer doesn't, ask him to order some for you.) Avoid dehydrated flavorings of substances rich in carbohydrates. Tomato paste is an example of these. But you can use stewed tomatoes, which are much richer in water content and so have a lower concentrate of carbohydrate.

As you read the recipes which follow, I'm sure you'll get an idea of both the variety and the types of dishes which you can eat.

## ROAST CHICKEN

1 chicken, 3 to 4 lbs.
⅛ lb. corn oil margarine

Season chicken with salt and place in roasting pan. Brush with melted margarine and add 1½ cups water to pan. Roast in 400° oven until browned. Then reduce heat to 300° and, basting frequently, continue to roast until breast meat is tender, about 20 to 30 minutes per pound. (Add more water when necessary.)

## POT ROAST

4 to 5 lbs. of beef (bottom round)
⅛ lb. corn oil margarine
1 cup water
1 can stewed tomatoes

Season meat with salt and pepper and let stand 15 minutes. Melt margarine in heavy deep pan, and brown meat on all sides. Add water and stewed tomatoes, cover tightly and simmer 2 to 2½ hours, or until tender when tested with a fork. (Add additional water when necessary.)

157

## FRIED CHICKEN

1 chicken, 3½ to 4 lbs.
several sprigs of parsley
3 stalks of celery
1 qt. water
¼ lb. corn oil margarine

Boil water, cut up chicken and place in boiling water with a little salt, parsley and celery. Simmer for 20 to 30 minutes. (During this time skim off fat.) Remove chicken from liquid and roll in gluten bread crumbs. Melt ¼ lb. of margarine in frying pan. Fry chicken over medium heat until well browned. Add more margarine if needed.

## FRIED CHICKEN LIVERS

1 lb. chicken livers
⅛ lb. corn oil margarine
gluten flour

Roll livers in gluten flour, melt margarine and fry livers over medium heat 3 to 5 minutes on each side, or until they are just pink, but not too done. Serve at once.

## FRIED EGGPLANT

1 eggplant
1 whole egg
¼ lb. corn oil margarine
gluten bread crumbs

Peel eggplant and cut into ½-inch slices. Melt margarine. Salt eggplant, dip into beaten egg and then roll in bread crumbs. Fry both sides over medium heat until well browned (about 5 to 7 minutes). Serve immediately.

158

## FRIED SHRIMP

1 lb. shrimp (raw)
¼ lb. corn oil margarine
gluten bread crumbs
1 whole egg

Clean shrimp. Dip into beaten egg and roll in bread crumbs. Melt margarine and fry shrimp until well browned, about 10 minutes.

## MUSHROOM SAUTÉ

1 lb. fresh mushrooms
⅛ lb. corn oil margarine
3 tbsp. sweet cream

Clean and slice mushrooms. Melt margarine and fry mushrooms for 5 to 10 minutes. Add ¼ cup of water and simmer for 5 minutes more. Then add cream and heat without boiling. Serve immediately.

## MUSHROOM OMELETTE

2 eggs
1 oz. safflower oil
¼ lb. mushrooms
2 tbsp. corn oil margarine

Clean and slice mushrooms and sauté in margarine for 5 minutes. Heat oil in frying pan. Beat 2 eggs, pour into oil and fry until eggs are set. Remove omelette to hot plate, place drained mushrooms in center, and fold omelette over.

159

## CHEESECAKE

2 level tsp. gelatin
¼ cup cold water
18 Sucaryl tablets
⅓ cup cold water

½ cup skimmed-milk powder
1 cup homogenized cottage cheese
2 tbsp. oil
2 tbsp. lemon juice
½ tsp. grated lemon rind

Soak the gelatin in cold water, add the Sucaryl tablets (crushed) and place over heat until gelatin and Sucaryl are dissolved. Beat together the cheese, oil, lemon juice and rind until smooth. Add ⅓ cup of water and ½ cup of skimmed-milk powder to the gelatin-Sucaryl mixture and beat with an electric mixer at high speed until stiff. Next fold this into the blended cheese mixture. Cover bottom of a small, oiled spring form (or flan ring) with a layer of cracker crust. Spread cheese cake mixture over crust and place in refrigerator for 4 or 5 hours to become firm.

This mixture may also be used as a pie filling with Gluten Nut Cracker Piecrust.

## GLUTEN NUT CRACKER PIECRUST

⅔ cup of crushed gluten nut crackers
⅓ cup wheat germ
1 tablespoon gluten flour
¼ cup safflower oil (or melted corn oil margarine)
1 teaspoon water in which 1 Sucaryl tablet has been dissolved

Crush crackers with rolling pin (an easy way is to place them between two layers of wax paper) and mix with wheat germ and flour. Beat oil or melted margarine and water together with fork. Stir this oil solution into cracker mixture, rubbing against the sides of the bowl until thoroughly mixed. It should be just moistened with the oil; if too thin add additional cracker crumbs. Spread and press mixture on sides and bottom of pie pan. Bake for 6 to 7 minutes in a slow oven (325°). Fill.

## CHAPTER TEN

# SOME CASE

# HISTORIES

AFTER I ARRIVED at my new nutrition principle
I put it into practice on a group of ninety-three obese
women. Every one who followed this nutritional pattern
lost weight. Over a year the losses ranged from 20 to
90 pounds. In every case there was a marked reduction in
body measurements, often quite out of proportion to the
weight actually lost, because these patients were losing
bulky fat, not relatively compact muscle tissue. Let me
tell you about some of these people. Perhaps you will
find some conditions similar to your own.

One woman, visiting my office for the first time, told
me that she had weighed 166 pounds two weeks before and
had not weighed herself since. During the two weeks she
had been following a standard diet. For breakfast she ate
one egg, a glass of orange juice, a slice of toast with jam,
and coffee with one lump of sugar. She skipped lunch. For
dinner she ate a small piece of meat or fish, smothered in
catsup, and again she drank coffee sweetened with one

lump of sugar. This regimen left her hungry, tired and occasionally dizzy. In addition, she had difficulty falling asleep.

When I put her on a scale, she noted, with shock, that she now weighed 174 pounds. In two weeks, *on a subnutritional pattern,* she had gained 12 pounds.

Her reaction was pure rage. She insisted first that my scale was inaccurate. There are two other scales in my office. Both confirmed her weight at 174 pounds.

"You've simply been eating too high a proportion of carbohydrates," I told her, "even though you haven't been eating enough over-all."

"I don't understand," she said.

I explained that the orange juice, toast, sugar and catsup were high in carbohydrate. I explained that skipping lunch was not helping, but hurting. With a good deal of enthusiasm, she switched to my new nutrition principle. Weight loss began immediately, and the side effects of her "low-calorie" program cleared up quickly, too.

Another woman, the wife of a physician, came to my office with a curious history. Not long before, she and her husband had joined friends at a well-known health resort, where everyone hoped to lose weight. She was the most obese person in the group. She had the highest hopes.

The regimen at the resort consisted of a diet ranging from 500 to 800 calories, but my future patient was specifically limited to 500 calories a day. After three weeks of diet, and considerable work with massage and exercise machines, three members of the group lost between 2 and

5 pounds. But the obese woman gained 12 pounds. This raised her weight to 188 and led the others to decide that she was cheating. Soon they worked out a plan to get evidence.

One day they had her called away from her room on a pretext and, while she was gone, turned her room inside out and upside down looking for hidden stores of food, much as one might search an alcoholic's room for hidden bottles. They found no hidden food, because there was none. When the physician's wife returned to her room she was furious. She packed her things, returned home and, in her anger, vowed she would never diet again, regardless of her appearance.

For the next month, indulging her appetite as she wished, she gained just one pound. Then, after meeting a patient of mine, she decided to come to my office.

Of course she was confused. "How could I possibly have gained more on a diet than I gained when I ate what I wanted to?" she asked.

It was a reasonable question. By eating what she liked, she had consumed a good deal of fat; by following a diet rich in salads, she had consumed a high proportion of carbohydrates. Neither she nor her physician husband had been aware that calories didn't count. When she adopted my principle and stepped up her calorie intake considerably, she began at once to lose weight.

I recall another patient who had weighed about 152 pounds for twenty years, but had never attempted to lose weight. "Why?" I asked her.

"Well, my husband is heavy, too," she said, "and he's always trying to lose weight and it just doesn't seem to work for him, so how could it work for me?"

"How does he try to lose?"

"Oh," she said, "with a new diet every six months. Ten years ago he weighed about ten pounds too much. Now he weighs about seventy-five pounds too much."

"Doesn't he ever lose weight?" I asked.

"Oh, yes," she said, "but he always gains it back. I think he's lost and regained about five hundred pounds since we were married."

After I explained the fallacies of the crash programs her husband had followed, this woman decided to try my new nutrition principle. Within a few months her weight dropped from 152 to 128, which is normal for her. This is important, but still more important, considering the background, is that at this writing the woman has maintained her weight loss easily for almost a year. She reports that her husband has resolved to follow her new nutrition pattern. Her great success seems to have been a challenge that he now wants to meet.

Into my office regularly come patients who are not just slightly obese. They are enormous. One 5-foot-6 housewife who came to see me weighed 210 pounds and had such a concentration of fat on her hands that she could not open and close them fully. Imagine what strain this put on the woman as she tried to hold her broom, make beds and wash dishes in the course of her household chores.

She believed that she was a compulsive eater. After the birth of her second child, she said, she had encountered some difficulty adjusting. Afterward, by her own description, she ate few meals, but she "nibbled ice cream, cake and candy all day." She complained of heartburn and fatigue. She was not happy in her girth and had tried a number of low-calorie diets. Two things always happened. She got dizzy and she cheated.

I will let her tell the rest in her own words:

"When I started the new program the first few weeks were hard. I was used to eating in a certain way and this new way was difficult to get used to. But in a week or so when I began to notice what was happening, the inches I was losing, I was delighted. I've been following the program now for fourteen months and once in a while I try to cheat a little just to see what happens. Do you know what happens? I get nauseated. I simply *can't* sit and nibble all day the way I used to. Now I have more energy than I can remember having. It used to be hard for me to take care of the children and to keep our apartment clean. Now I can turn the apartment upside down. I just feel better than I ever did."

This woman now wears a size 14 or 16 dress. Her weight is down 60 pounds, to 150. "I'm always taking in my dresses," she says. "The alterations cost so much that I decided to learn to sew myself."

A nurse whom I treated stood 5 feet 3 inches, weighed 160 pounds and wore a size 18 dress. Her eating was typical of obese people. She liked candies, cakes, ice cream, pizza pies. She had tried high-protein diets and low-calorie diets. Sometimes she managed to lose some weight, but these diets always left her exhausted. When she left the diets, she gained as much or more than she had lost.

In addition to eating carbohydrate, this nurse liked to drink them. She would drink as many as eight martinis some evenings. Often the total was lower, but martinis were a regular portion of her carbohydrate intake. She said she held her drinks well; she drank without getting very drunk. The martinis gave her a lift, but did not flatten her.

After I explained the new nutrition principle to her, she adopted it. "I'll get your weight down," I told her.

"I doubt it," she told me.

She followed the program religiously, and she no longer has doubts. Her weight, in a year, dropped 32 pounds to 128, and her dress size has shrunk to an 11. Does a size 11 dress on a 128-pound woman seem odd to you? To look at this nurse you would never guess that she weighed 128. By losing fat she lost more inches than she had thought possible. Now, at 128 pounds, she is actually lean.

Her drinking habits have changed, too. She now drinks safflower oil as enthusiastically as she once drank gin. Instead of vermouth she adds vinegar, and she says that she finds safflower oil and vinegar quite palatable. "I just can't seem to drink liquor any more," she says.

Certainly she is happier thin than she was fat. Perhaps

this has helped to control her drinking. But just as a high-fat diet tends to curb anyone's craving for carbohydrate food, so it seems possible that it can help curb a craving for high-carbohydrate drink. This is not, of course, sufficient evidence to recommend a high-fat diet as a treatment for excessive drinking. But in the case of this nurse the new nutrition principle was effective in a manner which I had not fully anticipated.

One slim, attractive housewife from a fashionable suburb of New York consulted me for an unusual reason. Her weight varied only between 101 pounds and 103 pounds and her figure gave her no problems. "But," she told me, "the only way I've managed to stay this way is to starve myself."

I asked her for her typical day's menu and here it is:

## BREAKFAST

Coffee (black)

## LUNCH

One peach
Coffee (black)

## DINNER

One portion of a green vegetable
One small piece of fish or meat
Coffee (black)

169

"How long have you been eating like this?" I asked her.

"For years. I don't remember exactly how long. But I'm hungry all the time. I can't remember not being hungry."

She switched to the new nutrition principle, and now, eating many times as much as formerly, she still weighs the same, still has her own trim figure. (Incidentally, her cholesterol level, which had been slightly elevated, came down.) Most significant to her is the fact that she no longer spends her days tormented by hunger.

One patient who, by my estimate, should lose roughly 85 pounds became concerned after she had lost 60. "I think I'm getting flabby," she said. I assured her that she was not, but the woman was convinced and a few days later visited one of the commercial slenderizing salons. She had read advertising claims about massage for many years.

At the salon, she was first given a tour of the machines and gadgets designed to help her lose. Then she was examined by the chief masseuse, who told her that she had to lose 25 pounds.

"Right now," the masseuse said, "your body is very firm. I feel it's only fair to warn you that if you lose the extra 25 pounds, you may develop some flabbiness."

"I haven't come here to lose weight," my patient said. "I've come here to lose flabbiness."

"But you aren't flabby," the masseuse said.

"I've already lost sixty pounds," my patient said.

170

The masseuse's answer was direct. "I don't believe you."

The woman returned to my office quite surprised. Even a masseuse, who presumably wanted the business, could not tell her she was flabby. So she now accepted my verdict as the truth. Further, the masseuse's inability to believe her weight loss convinced my patient that my new nutrition principle was more effective than any of the widely advertised commercial reducers.

A young resident physician in the hospital where I am an attending physician approached me with a vexing case. "A girl of seventeen," he told me, "who's suffering from obesity, among other things, just isn't responding to a low-calorie diet. Since she's in the hospital and in bed, we know she isn't cheating on food." (This, I must add, was quite some time ago, before my treatment for obesity had come to the formal attention of authorities at the hospital.)

"How many calories a day are you giving her?" I asked the resident.

"Only six hundred, and she keeps on gaining."

Any 600-calorie diet will have to be high in carbohydrate. The digestive tract needs bulk to function properly, and on so restricted a food intake the only way to provide that bulk is through carbohydrate. I placed the patient on my regimen, and, while bedridden, she not only stopped gaining, but lost 20 pounds. And, of course, while she lost she was eating many times 600 calories.

171

A woman patient of mine lost 25 pounds, but, with her weight down to a range of from 139 to 141, her reduction slowed. This happens sometimes. Occasionally weight loss will even come to a stop for a brief period.

"How long before I start losing again?" she asked.

"Soon," I said. "We'll cut your carbohydrate intake down a little further."

I could see she was disappointed that I could not promise her a 10-pound loss overnight. "There's a family affair next week," she said. "I hoped I could lose extra pounds."

"Your body is getting rid of excess fat as rapidly as it can," I pointed out.

The next time this woman visited me she was 7 pounds heavier. "What happened?" I asked.

"Oh, nothing," she said.

It took twenty minutes before I could get the truth out of her. Wanting to lose weight quickly, she had gone off her program and, instead of eating a lunch high in fat, she had switched to a commercial liquid preparation that advertises a low-caloric content. Whatever the caloric content may be, it is unimportant. This liquid preparation is rich in carbohydrate. Instead of eating meat or fish as her lunch staple, the lady switched to a "sure-fire" weight reducer, which triggered a complex chemical reaction and made her gain 7 pounds in a week. After that, she stuck to the new nutrition principle faithfully, and she has since lost the extra 7 pounds and more.

In order to obtain more evidence on the effect of poly-unsaturated fatty acids on heart ailments, I have organized an anticoronary club. The group meets regularly, and, while weight reduction is not its principal purpose, obese members have lost fat on my program.

One man, a successful dentist, had a 50-inch waist when he joined the club. He was, he explained, a compulsive eater and, compounding complications, he liked to drink. "Finishing a fifth of whiskey in one night is nothing for me," he said. Nor, I was to learn, was eating a loaf of bread, or two huge platters of spaghetti, plus an endless stream of between-meals snacks. I would say this man ate more than anyone I ever knew.

The dentist was not happy. His weight made him look years older, gave him leg pains and, with good reason, anxieties.

A patient walking into the dentist's office one day noticed a picture of a little boy. "Your grandchild?" he asked the dentist. It was, of course, the dentist's son.

A physician who knew the dentist once remarked to him, "The way you eat, you're a candidate for the pathologist's table. You're going to kill yourself. You'd better start drinking to keep your blood vessels dilated. Maybe that will put off the coronary for a while."

When the dentist drank he did not stop at one or two, as his physician friend had hoped. That was where the fifth a night came in. He drank hard and he drank glumly.

The new nutrition principle has revolutionized this

173

man's life. His waistline is down to 34 inches and he no longer drinks. "What's the sense of drinking?" he says. "I don't need it now."

One recent day a man he had treated at a resort some years ago walked into the dentist's office, stared at him a while and said, "Is your father a dentist? There's a dentist upstate who looks like you, but he's a lot older than you are."

The dentist's delight was boundless. By conquering his obesity, he said, he had grown younger by one full generation.

What about the dentist's compulsive eating? It continues and may still be continuing as you read this. But whatever he eats now is in accordance with the principle. "Extra slices of chicken?" he says. "No, I eat extra chickens." He eats as many as six veal cutlets at a sitting. (The cutlets are breaded with gluten crumbs and fried in corn-oil margarine.) He has found candies made without carbohydrates and he nibbles at them steadily. The dentist eats as much as he ever did, but he no longer bears the scars, outwardly or inwardly. He is now a well-built, stocky man. He was once enormous.

His case illustrates one important aspect of the principle as applied to compulsive eaters. The compulsion may remain, but by channeling it properly the eater does not harm himself.

I am reminded of some research work done among alcoholics on the Bowery. Each of the derelicts questioned

174

expressed a preference in drink. Some liked Scotch, some gin, some bourbon, some blended whiskey.

"Suppose you could switch," the interviewers said. "Suppose by drinking no more gin, but only Scotch, you could regain your dignity, your family, your job. Would you be able to do it?"

Almost to the man, the derelicts answered, "Yes, but I couldn't stop drinking."

The new nutrition principle does not ask compulsive eaters to stop eating. It asks only that they switch their foods and the method in which these foods are prepared. No one who follows the principle can possibly remain obese no matter how much he likes to eat and does eat.

Occasionally I encounter someone who is convinced that he or she is simply too fat to reduce. "I know your principle worked for others," they tell me, in effect, "but I'm pretty much of a hopeless case."

I remember specifically a 290-pound man I met in 1960. "My friends talk about your magic diet," he said, "but I'm afraid I'm beyond even magic."

I asked why he thought so.

"I can't remember not being heavy," he said. "It just must be hereditary."

"What are you doing about your weight?"

"Nothing now," he said, a little sadly. "Oh, I've tried things. I don't want to be heavy. When I've followed a diet I've followed it to the letter. Sometimes I lost, but only

175

temporarily. Once I lost forty pounds. But I was getting a little dizzy and so I had to stop the diet. Do you know what happened then?"

I could have guessed, but didn't.

"I not only regained the weight," the man said, "I came up with a bonus. I regained more than I had lost."

We talked longer and he mentioned the mental strain that always went with the diets he had tried. Half convinced that his obesity was hereditary, half convinced that a few more drastic dieting programs would shatter his mental equilibrium, this intelligent, successful man had given up.

I outlined my program for him and he set his goal at a weight loss of 100 pounds. Six months later, at this writing, the man was halfway there. He had lost 50 pounds.

"You know," he said, "when you outlined the diet I was surprised. I never heard of a diet that allowed cheese and fried foods." Then he told me how his surprise had turned to delight and how his attitude toward food had changed. He used to dread the dinner table; he no longer does. "I can't recall ever having felt so well, either physically or mentally," he said. His suit size has changed from 52 to 46.

What will your friends and relatives say about the new nutrition principle you are following? One of my patients encountered difficulty on this score. "We eat out a great deal," she said, "and it's quite a problem." She had not been having a successful time with the principle because

176

she had not been following it very well. "You see, I go somewhere and I pass up fruit juice," she said, "and the hostess asks why. When I tell her I'm on a diet she gets upset and says that I should start the diet somewhere else tomorrow, but not at her house tonight."

My advice on this score is simply to keep the principle to yourself for the first few weeks. This may mean curtailing your social activities, but passing up one or two dinner invitations is not very serious when viewed in perspective. Then, when the principle has worked changes in your shape, it will be easy to tell anyone you know what you are doing. No one will scoff at your new shape and so no one will scoff at the new principle you are following. In fact, people may very well want to find out about it themselves.

Accept my counsel and the experience of my patients on this score. Wait until you have been following the program for a short time before mentioning it. Then you will be walking proof that it works. You will not have to explain or convince anyone with words. You will convince them simply by your appearance.

Certain people suffer from unusual fat formation. We have all seen women with attractive figures that are spoiled by heavy legs. Since the new principle reduces excess fat, it enables you to lose from those areas where most fat is concentrated. If you are a victim of piano legs, you can expect your legs to show the most dramatic change under the program.

177

One woman I treated had an enormous fat formation on one arm. The other was much closer to normal. She had developed breast cancer some years earlier, and after the removal of a breast one arm accumulated so much fat that it was three inches larger in circumference than the other. No one can explain why this happened. Nothing revealed the cause and no treatment she tried had alleviated the condition. She always wore long-sleeved dresses.

As I considered, I must confess I had doubts. Since I could not be sure what had caused this strange fat formation, I could not be certain that the new nutrition principle would correct it. But since the principle is absolutely safe, I decided to try.

The patient lost fat generally, but lost most fat from the extra-heavy arm. Her figure is now close to normal and she now wears short-sleeved dresses.

Whatever the individual variations, these and all the other cases I have treated bear out the same point. The new nutrition principle gets rid of excess fat. Of course, there are differences from case to case—differences in the amount of carbohydrate I allow each patient, differences in the amount of oil I suggest each patient drink. Working with blood tests and a technical background, I can be more precise than you. But you, by applying common sense, can be precise enough.

Are you losing too slowly? Cut down on carbohydrate and increase the amount of oil you drink, if you can without becoming nauseated. Has your weight loss gone well

178

for a time, then suddenly stopped? Follow the same procedure.

Remember, what I have been outlining in this book is treatment for the "average" obese person. In whatever ways you vary from the average, you must compensate. Your own common sense will make such compensation simple.

There have been patients of mine who have had to stop eating *any* carbohydrate for a while. This is rare, but it is something you should know. You should realize, too, that such a regimen is temporary. For, as you lose fat, your tolerance for carbohydrates will increase. If you are inclined to obesity, you will probably never be able to eat large quantities of carbohydrates, but you will unquestionably be able to use some.

Bear in mind these two keys:

1. The more oil you drink, the more body fat you will burn.

2. The less carbohydrate you eat, the less body fat you will produce.

Apply the principle sensibly. Give your body months to rid itself of fat that has been acquired over years. This is not a "crash" program, but a safe program.

Your own feeling of health and your own rate of weight loss are indices. The new nutrition principle is your tool. Your own common sense, measuring each index, is what will make the tool work most effectively for you.

179

# CHAPTER ELEVEN

# THE END—AND
# THE BEGINNING

YOU HAVE BEFORE YOU the solution to your weight problem. This is as much as anyone else can do for you. Now you must begin to do things for yourself. If you are prompt in following my nutritional advice, you will be on the way to losing your extra fat in the time it has taken you to read this book.

Much of modern medical practice is based on the knowledge that each individual is unique. You may get colds frequently and mildly; your neighbor may get colds infrequently but heavily. Just as surely, your own obesity problem involves certain specifics which are part of your pattern of life. Someone else's obesity problem involves different specifics.

We now understand the general cause of most obesity conditions, and we understand how to counteract it. Only you can adopt the general treatment of a general condition to fit the specific individual, which you are.

A certain amount of mental discipline is necessary, but there is a certain amount of mental discipline in everything we do. We may not want to get up every morning, but we do when there is work to be done. We may not want to work at our desks on a sunny day when golf courses are beckoning. But we do, contenting ourselves with a promised round of golf on Sunday (when it rains).

There is a point where the mental discipline demanded by a program is too much for most people to endure. This alone was a strong argument against the low-calorie diets. We had to discipline ourselves unnaturally; we had to discipline ourselves to live with hunger in a land of plenty, to feel hungry and yet refrain from eating. I do not think that the mental discipline which my program imposes is in any way comparable. It is a small effort. We work when we would rather golf, and so we take a piece of cheese when we might prefer a chocolate sundae. I use "we" literally here. I have followed the principle myself for five years.

Understand that a great deal of what we do is habit. Eating patterns and appetite are habit, too. Hunger describes a very real thing: the body's demand for more food. But appetite is a habit we create. If you have an appetite for sweets, it is because you have created it. The body does not hunger for sweets, although many people have talked themselves into believing that it does. This principle will give you enough food to more than match your hunger. Usually it will curb your habit-formed appetite as well. But not always. Sometimes the appetite for more food than you need will persist. The answer for people who have prodigious appetites is to channel them properly so that the extra food will not be harmful, will not create obesity and will not shorten a normal life span.

Have you ever seen a thin person attack a steak with fury, then, with the steak two thirds eaten, suddenly stop? "It feels just like a curtain goes in front of my throat," one thin person told me, "and I simply don't want any more." He has satisfied his hunger. A fat man satisfies his hunger and then, instead of stopping, may go right on satisfying his appetite. No curtain drops for him. If he eats incorrectly, and probably he does, the fat man will move from weight plateau to weight plateau for all the rest of his life.

I say "probably" because most of us learned to eat improperly. We taught ourselves by satisfying our own individual tastes. Some of us like chocolate, some like vanilla, and we learned to eat accordingly. (We would be better off if we liked polyunsaturated fatty acids.) Our families influenced our eating. If your mother made a dish you liked years ago, you probably still like it now. You look for it in restaurants. If you are a woman you may like to make it yourself. If you are a man, you may ask your wife to make it.

Psychologists have shown that in some families food is an important means of obtaining both real and symbolic securities. Among American immigrant families, it has been learned, parents are particularly intent on stuffing their children, even to the extent of forcing them to eat far more than is necessary. Many parents in these families suffered starvation or deprivation before coming to the

United States. Without being aware of it, these parents are using food to build up their children against the racial or economic insecurity which plagued their own childhoods in "the old country."

Economics anywhere may have a large hand in the development of eating patterns. The play *Tobacco Road,* which had a record run on Broadway, told of a poor family in the American South which subsisted, almost exclusively it seemed, on turnips. Why? Because turnips were cheap and available. In other areas various cereals have been popular for the same reason. Carbohydrate food, generally, is cheaper than protein or the right kind of fat. Poor people eat carbohydrate, and even years later when they are no longer poor the habit continues. Eating habits formed in depression years persist into boom times.

Add up all the factors—background, tastes, environment, economics—and you can see that your diet is the sum total of your habits and the conditions of your life. Much is affected by the circumstances of your birth and the various factors in your environment. Food, we now know, is too important to be a matter of accident. You must teach yourself to eat properly, just as you once taught yourself to walk and to talk.

Neither your parents nor you yourself are to blame for your eating the wrong foods for many years. If they or you consulted nutrition experts, the answers probably were a bewildering mass of contradictory statements. There were fads and fallacies covering up facts, because until

183

now there simply wasn't much factual information on the cause and treatment of obesity. As a result, any nutrition fact that was discovered was emphasized beyond all reason.

The case of vitamins is an example. There is nothing wrong with vitamins, nothing wrong with "enriching" bread, nothing wrong with "fortifying" milk. But vitamins are only one aspect of a nutrition pattern. To get the most out of vitamins, you must take them in relation to other foods and according to your body's needs.

Since absorption of the fat-soluble vitamins, A, D, E and K, depends upon the presence of fat, it follows that those whose diet is deficient in fats may suffer from a deficiency of one or more of those essential vitamins as well.

Dr. Wallace F. Janssen, chief of public information for the U.S. Food and Drug Administration, recently had this to say about nutrition:

More people seem to believe more bunk about food and nutrition than about any other single topic in the health field and perhaps any other field. Today the old-time patent medicine man is back again, but this time he is a nutrition educator who tries to persuade you that a shotgun mixture of vitamins and minerals, plus some other secret factor not yet identified, is the answer to all health problems. This racket, probably the most widespread quackery in the United States, is estimated by the American Medical Association to be costing some ten million Americans 500 million dollars each year.

There is more to dieting than fads, than vitamins, than any other single consideration. In fact, the very word "diet" seems to have taken on unfortunate implications.

184

To many people it seems to imply weight reduction, or a hospital menu, restrictive and tasteless. The dictionary is kinder to the word. "Diet" comes from the Greek *diaita*, which means "a manner of living." And so diet involves not only food but attendant human values of conversation, companionship, and aesthetic satisfaction. It has been asserted, quite correctly, that when you tamper with a man's food you are tampering with the basic pattern of his life.

That is exactly what I am presuming to do, and I assure you it is not something I do lightly. But I know that if you are obese you are not happy with the existing basic pattern of your life. Almost all of us want to make a pleasing appearance, want to stay healthy, want to live long and useful lives.

I am trying to replace an unhappy pattern with a happy one. I am trying to replace bad habits with good. For in time, as you follow the new nutrition principle, the pattern itself will become a habit. The mental discipline I mentioned earlier will be less important. You will be eating correctly out of habit, just as for years you ate incorrectly out of habit. You may also find certain changes, for the better, in your over-all outlook.

One study of five hundred obese patients demonstrated that 93 per cent of them believed there was a connection between their emotions and their eating habits. If you overeat it is helpful to understand why you overeat. It is important, too, to understand that emotional factors may lead people to try to reduce when there is no physical reason why they should. We have, necessarily, stressed

185

obesity, but I want to mention, too, that if your weight is now satisfactory you should leave it that way. Don't think that a 10-pound loss from normal weight will help your appearance or outlook. My principle will not get you down below normal weight, but crash programs will. You should not lose any more fat than the principle enables you to lose. If you are heavy-boned and broad-beamed, there is nothing you can do to become small-boned and thin as a rail. If you try, you will be endangering yourself. I mention one case cited by an eminent psychologist.

A girl twelve and a half years old was admitted to a hospital after her weight dropped from 98 to 53 pounds. She had been starving herself. This had been a pretty girl, slightly obese at 98 pounds, but not seriously so. Taunting children at school suggested that she diet because she was fat and unattractive. Then a friendly boy turned his attentions away from her and toward a girl who lived nearby. In a neighborhood quarrel that followed, the chubby girl's father was severely beaten by relatives of the second girl.

This last event assumed great importance because the chubby girl lost some respect for her father and the father lost some respect for himself. Afterward the chubby girl, who did not really have to lose weight, who actually was pleasingly plump, began to starve herself, to such an extent that she became cadaverous and was taken to a hospital. (The story has a happy ending. After therapists worked with the girl and her parent, the family regained its self-respect and the girl ate normally again.) It is my hope that no one of normal weight, no one who does not need to reduce, concludes from this book, "the thinner the better." A conclusion like that is as erroneous as "the fatter the better." A body functions best when it contains 11.3 per cent fat. Large variations *either* way are harmful.

Psychologists have done a great number of studies on obesity. Some maintain that an enlarged body is the fat person's defense against a hostile world. Symbolically, they say, the fat man sees in his very fat a defense against a world which seems against him. Medically we know that the fat, instead of being a defense, is in itself a threat.

Others have found in cases of obese sterile women that the fat represents a symbol of the pregnancy the woman so badly wants. She cannot actually become pregnant, so, unconsciously, she compromises by trying to shape her body into the form of a pregnant woman. Actually, the extra fat decreases whatever chance she has, however small, of finding a cure for her infertility.

Still others have correlated sexual inhibition and maladjustment with obesity. The woman is afraid of men, afraid of the sexual experiences men will want. By becoming gross, she discourages male attention, not in the complicated series of maneuvers that a beautiful woman who is fearful of sex must undergo. She stops the maneuvers before they start by becoming so obese that men are not inclined to start them.

There is even evidence that many innately lazy people

187

grow fat so that they will have a convenient excuse for laziness. This goes a little deeper. The belief of many psychologists is that lazy people, people who are under-active, are fearful of undertaking activities. An anxiety is at the root of the laziness and the laziness is at the root of the obesity.

Perhaps the most common psychological pattern in obesity is the one in which an individual eats when feel-ing low, to cheer his spirits. Eating in itself is satisfying, even to people who are perfectly normal. The depressed neurotic finds heightened satisfaction in eating and so eats on and on.

I am not a psychiatrist and I do not attempt here to prescribe for any emotional causes that may have con-tributed toward your obesity. If obesity is a symptom of a disturbance, I can treat the symptom. The new principle will eliminate it. But if the emotional disturbance is seri-ous and exists independent of the obesity, then the situa-tion is beyond my province.

There is a point I am qualified to make, though, to people who eat whenever they feel depressed. This is a habit, and although by following the new principle you can eat unlimited quantities, it would be sorry use of my research if you used it to justify hoggishness.

We all get depressed at times, sometimes with good reason and sometimes without any reason that we know. But there are many other means than eating to defend yourself against a depressive state. Instead of oral intake, such as eating, try visual intakes. Reading, watching television or movies are visual intakes. You can condition yourself to turn to a hobby when the depressive mood is upon you. Hunting, golf, card playing, sailing, bowling—there are dozens.

To me, an excuse that you cannot lose weight because you are emotionally upset simply does not stand up. Unless you are suffering from a serious mental disturbance—a fractional proportion of fat people are in this category—you can exert the discipline you need to change your eating habits so that your diet falls within the framework of my principle.

I have treated obese people in sufficient numbers to know that they can find as many excuses for being fat as an alcoholic can find for being drunk. These excuses, in the main, are valueless, whether they are used to conceal truth from a physician or to conceal truth from yourself. There is no longer any excuse for staying obese except inertia. And if your own appearance and the handicaps you suffer from obesity are not convincing enough to make you want to lose your excess fat, I hope the hazards of obesity which I mentioned are.

We can go back to William Banting for a description of what obesity meant to one man. A century ago, after the high-fat diet had worked so sucessfully for him, Banting wrote:

Of all the parasites that affect humanity I do not know of, nor can I imagine any more distressing than that of obesity, and having just emerged from a very long probation in this affliction, I am desirous of circulating my humble knowledge and experience for the benefit of my fellow man with the earnest hope that it may lead to the same comfort and happiness I now feel under the extraordinary change—which might almost be termed miraculous had it not been accomplished by the most simple common-sense means.

A long sentence indeed, a sentence from another time, and yet one which to me is quite touching. It states some of my own feelings and describes some of my own experience. Banting, in his day, went as far as he could. He could not perfect his dietary pattern or advance further than he did, because in his time the physiology of obesity was one more mystery as yet unsolved by advancing medical science.

Today we have solved much of the mystery, but some of Banting's words still apply. Eating properly and maintaining a normal weight can be "accomplished by the most simple common-sense means." In this book the means have been presented to you. The common sense, I'm quite sure, you already have. It is now up to you to bring the two to work on the single problem of obesity.

This is the end of my book. It can be the beginning of a new life for you.